Uncorking a Wonderful Life

My Path from Drunk to Sober

Bob Schober

ISBN: 9780578853482

Cover photo by © Rene Laventure
Book design by © Amanda Costello

First printing edition 2021

*To my wife Rene for her constant love and support,
and to Sierra, my stepdaughter, for teasing me about my faults.*

Acknowledgements

I owe a huge debt to my longtime and very dear friends Emanuel B., Nona M., Tom D., Ron L., and Jim and Kay K. and the hundreds of folks who shared their stories, kicked me in the butt and encouraged me to seek a life of sobriety.

My deep thanks to Tom B., Randy S., John R., Mauno S., Kathryn F., Jim M. and Nancy N. who read this book and gave me their loving insights to make this book that much better. And thanks to Kendra L., for polishing the manuscript.

CONTENTS

Introduction

He jolted awake. Not from the deep sleep of the untroubled but from another booze-soaked coma. Head pounding, mouth dry as dust, stomach acid searing his throat, he slowly came afloat in a sea of aches, eyes swollen, lips chapped. He groaned in fear: Where the hell am I? It took a moment for his eyes to focus and he realized he was home in his bedroom; sheets, quilt and clothes tangled on the floor. He half rolled over to find that this time, thank God, there was no one in bed with him. He tried to dredge up last night but his memory, clouded by alcohol, slowly replayed some of the verbal brawls, bullying, the chastising of his mates for not drinking enough, and then ... blank. He couldn't remember anything past that shot of whatever. He did remember walking into the bar, giving his car keys to the owner and telling him that under no circumstances, no matter how much he argued or begged, to give those keys back to him. He did remember what he usually did at night's end: "Gimme those fucking keys or I'll bust your head."

He felt awful as always, his mind full of dread. How the hell did I get here? Slowly, nauseously, he crawled to the window and pulled the curtain back. His car sat at the curb, not on the lawn this time, and, with heart pounding, he squinted at his fender. There were no new dents, blood, or scraps of clothing he could see. "At least I didn't kill anyone," he mumbled and fell back into bed.

That guy was me. That was my world. Drinking was my security, delusion my reality. I was crazy. Suicidal. A miracle saved me.

I am an alcoholic. It's the central fact of my life. Addiction to alcohol and assorted character flaws conspired to consume my morality and sense of self. My childhood carefree love of the outdoors where I danced with the sun, wind, trees, birds and flowers died in family tragedy. I was a lost child when alcohol found me. This book is my story of recovering from the ravages of drinking and getting sober. I started my journey, when near to drinking myself to death, I was saved by a miracle that opened my eyes, and I chose to be sober. I haven't had a drink of alcohol for thirty-five years, which has made possible a life more wonderful than I ever dreamed possible.

In these pages I will tell you how that happened. You'll read about why I started drinking, how I stopped, and the path I followed to achieve sobriety. You'll read how I had to change everything I could about how I thought, how I acted in the world, and what I believed in. The first and most important thing I had to do was stop looking at the world through the bottom of a glass.

Desperate drinking proved how deeply I had fallen into spiritual despair. I drank like a thirsty horse at a desert trough and had created the persona of a long-nosed prig cloaked in self-righteous bravado, who judged the flaws of others to hide my own failures. To salve my own feelings of inadequacy, I tried to tear others down to my level, which I believed was as a nothing.

My real problem was me. I was a child in a man's body, emotionally stuck at age twelve when I had my first drink. I didn't know how to deal with the grief and hard knocks that seemed to follow me, so I puffed up with liquid courage to maintain my image of not giving a damn about anything. In reality, I was scared shitless about almost everything and everyone. (See Note 5 for reasons people use drugs and alcohol.)

To survive past the age of thirty-seven, I had to stop boozing. There was a problem, however: denial. I wasn't an alcoholic, you see, because I could stop whenever I wanted to. I just didn't want to until the day I knew I had to.

Plugging the jug is the single, most important thing I have ever done, but I didn't realize how important at the time. My world had shrunk into a bottle, and all I had left before I quit was more drinking. All I wanted was drinking. I sacrificed my wonder and curiosity for booze.

Stopping proved to be the lowest hurdle in a field of high-bar emotional degradations and denials. Change came slowly for me because of my fear and stubbornness at giving up what I knew. The promise of a changed life lured me to tackle the hard inside work; I had to purge my mind of self-told lies and cleanse my heart of the anger and secrets that were key drivers of my drinking and bad behavior. I struggled with that work, but my willingness to clear out the muck opened a path to a new life. To get there, I also had to accept that I can never conquer my addiction to alcohol – it's a disease of the spirit etched in my heart. I learned how to keep my active addiction in remission through nourishing my love of living by changing how I think about myself and act towards others.

***

I thought for years about writing this story but always found an excuse or two to put it off. Too busy, nobody would care -- you get the picture. But lately some long-buried grief and fits of anger and impatience kept popping up, and I knew I had to write about my drunk and sober lives to better understand what those feelings were really about. I discovered more about myself than I expected.

It's taken me a year to write it all down. The actual writing itself, and grasping for the right words, uncovered an even greater sense of the fears, beliefs, and buried emotions I felt as a child and still struggle with as an adult.

Writing certain sections of the book was difficult. I had to time-travel my gut and mind back to my younger years and feel again the abandonment and fear that haunted me then. In other sections I had to get much more honest about the real cause – me – in my troubles with my father, brother, and others. Some of my portrayals of this journey may seem a little over-drawn, as I often failed to find words adequate to convey the powerful emotions that ruled me at the time. Words like "terror" and "love" hardly capture the totality of what I felt in some moments, but I've written these emotional scenes as truthfully as I could.

The writing helped me get to a deeper understanding of what drinking cost me and what I inflicted on others. I drilled down into other dark corners and discovered some long-buried history that I'll tell you about. I uncovered a long-buried, never-to-be-remembered grief over my mother's death that's helped me understand the true relationships I had with my father, brother, and sister and people in general.

***

Addiction is a territory for which only those of us who live in it can truly know the cruel desperation and pain that lurks there. And only addicts like me who find sobriety, no matter the type of addiction, truly know the fabulous joy in finally touching the happiness and emotional freedom we all yearned for. For me it felt like I had been starved and suddenly found nourishment.

My story is a small corner of that land, and I leave it to readers to reflect on my story through the prism of their own life experience.

I believe that addiction of any kind is an incurable, chronic disease – but treatable. I think that the road to addiction is like falling into a hole and grabbing a shovel to dig your way out. Many just keep digging deeper, but I was lucky -- someone jumped in with a ladder and helped to pull me out.

Sobriety is an intensely personal journey, a solo dive-deep inside to confront our fears and pry out our secrets. Some resist taking that road so strongly that they go back out. Relapse is common for any addiction and can be part of the process of recovery. There is an upside. Many organizations and people all over the world are ready to help anyone to achieve recovery, and they welcome back those who relapse. (See Note 8 for addiction statistics and Note 3 for sobriety success statistics.)

This book is also for those of you worried and confused about what's happened to your loved ones who may be wallowing in a dead-end disaster of addiction. I hope my story can help them to recognize similar emotional and physical whirlwinds that may have affected their friends or relatives. Understanding the past is the first step in healing.

I've been around recovering men and women of all backgrounds and personal hells long enough to know that no matter how our childhoods differed, we all tend to react the same way -- by burying painful memories deep inside and grasping for alcohol, drugs, food, sex, gambling, weight-lifting—anything at all to dull the pain. A search for relief can lead to bizarre places and desperate ends. (See Note 5 for research results on why people use.)

"An abnormal reaction to an abnormal circumstance is normal behavior," Holocaust survivor Victor Frankl wrote in Man's Search for Meaning.

You may find my family background different from your own, and that's no surprise. No two stories are alike. Many have had childhoods far worse than mine.

I had a very full but sheltered childhood. I never suffered from beatings, sexual abuse, physical neglect, or alcohol/drug addled parents. I always had plenty to eat, clothes to wear, new shoes, and bicycles and baseball mitts when I needed or wanted them. My parents and sister doted on me when I was a toddler, encouraged me to read and study hard in school. Dad had money for college, which conveniently gave me a pass on the Viet Nam War.

Maybe you'll read about my privileged upbringing and think I was just a pansy-assed spoiled kid who threw a tantrum because his silver spoon went missing. You'd be right to ask, "You had everything I never had so how could you possibly understand what I've gone through?" I can't possibly know. But I can guess.

I've heard hundreds of recovering people share stories of childhood desperation and pain, and from their honesty and courage, I've come to believe that addicts share one thing in common. Most of us, regardless of upbringing, suffered some childhood trauma of personal loss, possibly severe, repeated physical or mental abuse, or, in my case, a fear of abandonment. No matter the cause, such trauma causes intense pain which fuses into anger, fear, resentment, demoralization, and low self-esteem in a desperate search for relief.

Even so, I can't fully comprehend any story other than my own, so I don't presume to tell anyone what they need to do about their personal past. You know your own addiction history, and I share mine in this book so you can know me a little. This book is my personal history of my own trauma that defined my drinking life.

I think it's obvious that all addicts live in their own personal hells, but I believe the details don't really matter. We all begin recovery from the same spiritually dead place, and need to scrounge up whatever commitment and perseverance we have the strength to muster to find sobriety.

***

This book is not a "drunk-a-log" detailing my boozing escapades. Other authors have written about that more than I think helpful. I've written this book as an outline--or better yet, as a map of my trail from addiction to recovery that I hope may help some readers chart their own journey.

It is also not a "how to" manual. There is no big "T" of truth in these pages other than "abstinence is the launch code for recovery" (my words). There is a small "t" that is my own truth that I need to feel, grieve, and atone for.

There is, however, a capital "I," something: getting and staying sober was absolutely the most important, demanding, and life-saving journey I will ever make. It wasn't a sashay along smooth ground, either; bouldering around my denials finally helped me exhume my long-lost sense of commitment, regain faith in what I was doing, and strengthen my will to keep to the path. I needed all of that to stay steady amid the emotional ups and downs along the way.

I also want to emphasize that there is no One Way, one Golden Path into sobriety. I found sobriety in Alcoholics Anonymous (AA), but there are other places where you can look. AA has some religious and spiritual overtones which turn some people off (it did me at first). (See Note 1 for information on AA.)

Other recovery groups teach abstinence maintenance from a more secular base without religious or spiritual overtones. No matter which type of group you choose, they all share a common goal – staying sober. It's the only thing that really matters. (See Note 2 for information on secular groups.)

***

Some members of AA may argue that by writing about my experience in AA, I've broken my anonymity, which undermines AA's core principle that urges members to keep their anonymity in public and with each other to "place principles before personalities."

Bill Wilson wrote these 12 Traditions in 1946, a time when alcoholism carried such a strong stigma that anonymity was a critical shelter for those trying to stay sober. I argue that today, alcohol and drug addiction is so public and prevalent a societal problem that talking about it gives great benefit. Knowledge is power, as the saying goes, and I believe the more everyone knows about the risks of addiction and ways to move away from it, the more sufferers can get help. (See the sidebar on page 25 to read the 12 Traditions.)

The principle of anonymity, however, is crucial to the success of the AA program. Most addicts, including me, come to their first meeting as egomaniacs encrusted in low self-esteem. Every group has a wide assortment of people with different backgrounds, and the beauty of it all is that taking a seat makes everyone equal. There is no caste system.

To honor the spirit of the tradition of anonymity, I use no last names in the book, even though some of my sober friends voiced no objection to my using them. It's my small way of honoring the spirit of the Traditions. I don't promote what I did, and I hope my story attracts others enough to launch their own journeys.

***

I've organized this book in two parts. Part I focuses on how my drinking life started and what compelled me to stop. I share about my family, the fears and terrors that grew inside me, and how I got sober in Alcoholics Anonymous and in-house treatment.

Part II tells of my struggles with the 12 Steps, the work I did to achieve emotional sobriety, and the issues I still need to work on. In later chapters I share about the healing work going on with my brother and uncovering some unresolved grief that I still need to work with. That work healed my mind and soul.

The Notes at the end of the book provide detailed information and research summaries on a variety of subjects, including why people use, the addict brain, grief, sobriety statistics, the effects of alcohol on the mind and body and more. I've also included a list of books that helped me better understand where I came from and where I'm headed.

PART I:
DARK to DAWN

First you take a drink, then the drink takes a drink,
then the drink takes you.
--F. Scott Fitzgerald

A man could get drunk, then there was no loneliness, for a man
could people his brain with friends, and he could find his
enemies and destroy them.
--John Steinbeck, The Grapes of Wrath

I begin this story on a cold, misty Pacific Northwest winter day in Bellingham, Washington, in November 2019. At noon I walked into my regular AA meeting room near the seashore and helped myself to a cup of lousy coffee. Strong, bitter tasting coffee seems to be an AA tradition that keeps me alert for the hour-long meeting. I took a seat in my regular place next to some of my buddies and looked out a window to see the trees waving in the wind.

I shook hands with my friends, introduced myself to others I didn't know, and chit-chatted until the chairperson called the meeting to order. I was excited, because I knew the chairperson would ask, "Does anyone have a birthday in the current month that wishes to be recognized?" When the question came, I raised my hand.

"On November 2, I, Bob S., reached thirty-five years of continuous sobriety, one day at a time." (It's common not to use a last name in honor of an anonymity tradition).

To cheers, applause, handshakes, and hugs, I received my AA coin and sat back down with tears gathering in my eyes. Once again, I felt so grateful to be sober, and that guides appeared with a ladder when they did so I could enjoy that moment.

I wondered, as I half-listened to others speak to the topic of the day, how did my drinking start? Why did I turn into the warped, fearful man I became? What paths did I travel to become the man I am now? The clues point back to when I was a kid.

CHAPTER 1
WHAT HAPPENED?

*As an alcoholic, you will violate your standards quicker
than you can lower them.*
--Robin Williams (Yes, that Robin Williams)

*Nothing is any particular way. It's your state of mind
that creates reality.*
--Frederick Lenz, Zen teacher

Tragedies happened.

I entered this world chubby and cheerful (just over ten pounds), with wide eyes and a smile to match. My great-aunt Flora always told me I was the happiest baby she had ever seen. Family pictures show me in a highchair laughing and coddling a doll or sitting entranced by the ornaments and tinsel reflecting a kaleidoscope of colored lights on our Christmas tree.

Nature's beauty, vastness, and strangeness enchanted me. I'd lay on our front lawn imagining castles in the sky and then build those castles in my sandbox; and I'd sit on my swing and hurl myself toward the sky.

On other days my friends and I spun around dizzily and flopped on the grass, or we just tumbled and wrestled with abandon. We liked to race around the block and to go explore in the bushes at the park. In the evening I'd toss and softball back and forth with a friend or play Red Light, Green Light with all the neighborhood kids. It was all just fun, and every day I laughed more than I cried.

I loved sunlight and thunder, music and laughter, trees and flowers, blue sky and scudding clouds. I loved being read to by

1

my mother and paged through encyclopedias before I could read. I fondly remember sitting in Grandpa Wall's lap (my mother's father) as he read Peter Rabbit and Uncle Wiggly stories while Grandma Cora set mountainous lemon meringue pies on window-sills to cool.

My childhood was truly idyllic. But not for long. I was eight years old when three of my grandparents passed away in 1956 and 1957. Mom's parents, Wall and Cora, died of heart attacks, and Dad's father Gallus died from Lou Gehrig's disease. I remember reading stories to Grandpa Gal as he lay immobile in bed wasting away. I remember crying at their funerals. But there was an earlier tragedy.

My older brother Don and I shared an upstairs bedroom in our house. One morning, when I was seven and he was thirteen, he woke up and couldn't swallow. The family doctor diagnosed polio, a scary, deadly disease in the early 1950s with no vaccine.

Dad and Mom rushed him to the hospital, came back home. Mom cried as Dad told my sister Peg, then eleven, and me, "Your brother's in the hospital and could die." They turned to enter their bedroom and closed the door. Peg started to cry and rushed into her bedroom and closed the door. I didn't know what "could die" meant, but I was suddenly alone and really scared. I don't remember what I did after that. Maybe I ran upstairs to my bedroom and cried or rushed outside to be with the trees. I was shocked.

I do remember that Peg and I were kept home from school in quarantine, and sometime later that year we took the sugar cube doused with the Salk vaccine. I remember having to stay alone in the car during family visits to Don because I was too young to be allowed in the hospital. With my brother gone, going upstairs to bed became very scary. Don survived, and months later, he came back home. Everything changed when he walked back in the door.

Dad and Mom understandably took special care with Don,

hovering over him in fear he might have suffered other damage from his hospital stay. Their entire focus was on him, and I, of course, was too young to understand what was going on. I still wanted and needed to be coddled, and this sudden shift left me feeling left out and, once more, alone. I blamed Dad and Mom – and became angry and jealous of Don, too – for what I thought was pushing me aside.

And then three years later when I was ten, Mom died from cancer. Her death was a catastrophe that exploded the veneer of family normalcy. None of us – Don, Peg, or me – knew how seriously she was in danger of dying. Dad never talked with us about that. I know now that his aim was to protect us, but the sudden shock only devastated us.

I remember that when Dad told us, Don and Peg cried, and I got angry. I rushed out of the room furious and started throwing things at a kitchen wall. I felt betrayed and suddenly abandoned. I soon began to feel "survivor's guilt," ashamed of myself for not knowing she was sick or doing something to help her.

After Mom's death I turned from happy to angry, hopeful to confused, confident to desperate. I was just a kid and didn't really understand my emotions, but I turned to a vision of myself as an unworthy kid and, despite doing the "right" things, a fraud. No matter my good grades in school or activities in church and Boy Scouts, I was a walking-talking, two-legged lie.

Dad was crushed, also, and probably couldn't talk with us about Mom's death. But he even went so far as to prohibit us from talking about Mom's death with anyone outside the family. I don't remember him ever trying to console me. Dad remarried a year later, filling his own need and Ruth, bless her heart, turned out to be a wonderful and doting stepmother and, I believe, saved our family.

Mom's death shattered me and the life I knew, so I created a new world to hide in where my anger and fears festered. In that fantasy world I created stories to explain what happened. I blamed Dad, and for some reason, I blamed myself for her dying. I told myself this story over and over until it became smooth, like a stone in my hand worn smooth by water, and I flung it at every problem that came my way.

Family pictures show me at the time as a brow-furrowed, unhappy looking kid who needed help. I wanted something—anything for my pain, and I yearned for relief. I found it two years later and fell head-over-heels in love with it.

CHAPTER 2
THE DAY I FELL IN LOVE

Whiskey is liquid sunshine.
--George Bernard Shaw

It started with a sip.

My family was of German background, and we sometimes spoke Deutsch at home. We celebrated Christmas with German carols and toasted holidays with sweet German wines. Thinking it's better for kids to taste the stuff at home than away, Dad sometimes let my toddler lips sip from his glass. I later graduated to my own glass and fell in love with the taste and sensation. I always begged for just a little bit more, please, please, but Dad usually said no. He often put out liqueurs for ice cream, though, and let me pour them on.

In the summer of 1960, I was twelve, and Mom had been dead for two years. It was a typical Milwaukee summer day in July–ninety degrees and sticky, as I pushed the hand mower lathered in sweat. Thirsty, I went inside for some milk or soda, when suddenly, I had a first-time ever thought – I'll make a drink! The clock read after 2 p.m., but it was High Noon for me. I was about to dive into a deep hole that would imprison me for the next twenty-five years.

I always seemed acutely aware when alcohol was around. I closely watched as my stepmother Ruth mixed a drink for herself (she was not an alcoholic), and watched Dad bartend for their friends (he wasn't either). The social ritual of drinking intrigued me. I watched the adults mix a cocktail with a flourish, and joke as they cradled a glass; their rolling laughs and slurred speech filled the room with a sense of intimacy and well-being. I wanted that, too.

I was really excited. I closed the refrigerator door and opened the recycled in-wall ironing board cabinet that Dad had made to store the liquor bottles. A family taboo hung in the air, but I blew it off. I knew I had to do this right – and not get caught. I grabbed a bottle of Fleischmann vodka and instinctively noted how the bottle sat on the shelf – if there was any question that addiction was in my blood, this confirmed that there was. After all, so-called "normie" people don't pay that kind of attention to their liquor bottles.

I dumped ice cubes in a tall glass, filled it more than halfway with vodka, and topped it off with tonic water. I chugged it as I would a cold soda and put the bottle back with the label set exactly as before.

I went back to mowing the lawn when … Wow! I felt woozy, as if I was flying in a cloud that stilled my squirreling mind. I want more of that! I of course beelined back inside. This time I made sure to grab a different bottle. Canadian Club sounded tasty. I filled a glass with ice, poured until half full, topped it with ginger ale and chugged the whole glass. I put the CC back as I had found it.

How much booze had I consumed? I guess about ten ounces, all within twenty minutes or so. A harbinger of my future.

I went outside again, my mind blown wide open. I felt weightless and danced to a new music flooding through my mind. I laughed and fell on the grass and rolled around. I had found what I needed! For the first time in a couple years, I felt GOOD and HAPPY. Somehow, some way, I finished mowing the lawn.

I don't remember making a third drink, but I passed out in the sunroom recliner. I didn't come to until Dad and Ruth got home from work. They must have been surprised to see me napping in the chair, because I was NEVER inside the house when they got home. I was usually in the nearby park playing tennis, or hitting fly balls, or doing anything to stay outside and away from home. I must also have reeked of alcohol, but neither of them said a word. In a nanosecond I knew I could get away with doing a lot more tasting if I was careful.

Over the following days and weeks, I investigated all the other bottles in that cabinet. There must have been a dozen different brands of gin, vodka, bourbon, whiskey, scotch and more. I helped myself to them all, always making sure to align them on the shelf as they had been, and not taking too much to be noticeable. I sometimes added water to my favorites just to be sure no one would notice.

I started feeding drinks to my friends whenever Dad and Ruth went out for the night. I'd invite them over to play cards and I'd bartend. I grew pretty proficient at cocktailing, making drinks that I had learned by watching Dad bartend for family friends. How proud I felt! I was a better drinker than them!

I often wanted to drink. I soon *needed* to drink, and I needed my friends to join me. I was uneasy about stealing the booze, so to ease my conscience I roped in my friends – I wasn't the only one supplying drinks, so that made it okay. At bottom, however, I really didn't give a damn. Drinking gave me something to be proud of. It didn't salve my loneliness.

CHAPTER 3
MY EXTERIOR

All that glitters is not gold.
Shakespeare, The Merchant of Venice

I started out as an intelligent young man full of promise, blessed with an outgoing personality and a love of the outdoors and books. I had all the advantages of a white, upper-middle class upbringing in the 1950s and '60s – good schools, great teachers, and a safe neighborhood with a park a half block away to play in. I was taught that obeying the rules and being a good boy would bring the brass ring in reach and bestow the success promised to hard-working, well-to-do white men. The future was my oyster, as the saying goes.

It was a fantasy. Hope died.

In my early teens, I became obsessed with finding answers: Why had Mom died? Why didn't Dad tell me she was dying? Does Dad still love me? Why am I such a loser? Why don't things work out for me as they do for others? What the hell is going on?

I continually asked myself those questions, but no one could help me find the answers. I grew angrier and more desperate not knowing where I was, what was real, and where I was going. Life became a threat, not a promise.

Anger can't be sealed away; it will always leak out, quietly with passive-aggressiveness or explosively with fists. It did that with me after Mom's death and only got worse.

I would suddenly lash out with words when a friend wouldn't do what I wanted. Or with my fists when really triggered. One time when I was about twelve, a blocked football pass bloodied and almost broke my nose. I flew into an instant fury, threw a fist and knocked out my friend. I would punch someone for no reason

8

and then, feeling ashamed about what I had just done, would beg them to hit me back. I flipped anger and shame like pancakes on a hot griddle.

My fear of other people deepened in high school, and I began to isolate. I thought that standing apart from personal connections would protect me from being found out as the fraud and failure I believed I was. In those four years I never once went to the cafeteria for lunch. I went on only one date and never attended dances, including the junior and senior proms. I moved myself to the edge and looked at everything as through a side window.

I made myself a victim to explain what wasn't going right for me. It was everyone else's doing because I certainly wasn't at fault. To punish those assholes – I'll show you! -- I began to isolate myself from others, especially those I thought were smarter, stronger, or better looking.

I emotionally split into two personas like opposite sides of a coin – I could flip a happy face to cover my emotional sullenness. The tension became too great; I was like a chunk of matter cozying up to antimatter. Explosive emotions were the result.

I could back slap and laugh with the best of them when playing sports or going to the movies with friends; then changing on a dime, I would slash them with ridicule for their flaws. At times I would burst into anger over a slight, but I realize in hindsight that I acted that way to keep others off-balance to shield my own vulnerabilities. I was like a jack-in-the-box, humming a tune and getting along with an asshole waiting to pop up, and some days it was a guess which one would show up.

My self-image eroding, masks became my specialty defense. I could walk into a room full of people and, like a chameleon, instantly flip personas to manipulate their impressions of me. In a crowded room I would be suave and literate with folks I wanted to impress, and become a cussing, foul joke-telling boor with the

9

group I wanted to be accepted by. I had little sense of myself, so I had to keep the illusions going.

I don't want to give the impression that I was emasculated by depression. Many things continued to give me pleasure – sports of many kinds, including golf, tennis, and softball; the game of Risk, a good movie. But once the games ended, my morose guy took over.

In English class I read the story of Sisyphus in Greek mythology. Zeus, the head god, damned Sisyphus to hell, where Hades condemned him for eternity to roll a huge boulder up a hill, only for it to roll down when it neared the top. I identified with him immediately – it seemed that no matter how hard I tried, I always ended back in the same place – alone, frustrated and angry. I created my own Catch-22: the more I believed I was a failure, the less I risked, and the more I stayed stuck, the more frustrated I became.

I was becoming delusional. Despite my deepening frustration and confusion about who I was, I still needed affirmation. Since I believed I was a nothing, the only way to get positive attention was to shape-shift.

I was still young enough to think that following in my brother's and father's footsteps would make me a somebody in the family. I needed to be a scientist, just like them. Don earned a Ph.D. in chemistry and Dad was a graduate mechanical engineer. I was drawn to astronomy. The night sky and stars amazed me, and I spent many a freezing winter night peering through our telescope on the upper rear porch.

My interest in the stars convinced me that I could be an astrophysicist, a vainglorious idea built on my skills with addition, long division, and algebra. The name itself –astrophysics – sounded more prestigious than mere chemistry or engineering. The subject was out of this world, so to speak, just where I wanted to be. I envisioned myself robed in stars and equations and strutting before my peers like I knew something they didn't.

I played this fantasy out in my junior and senior years by carrying astrophysics texts with an armload of other schoolbooks. I of course showed off the front cover to attract some oohs and aahs – Gee, how smart you are! I also thought those texts haloed me with a "coolness" that melted *theirs*. It also was my way of sneering at those dunderheaded footballers, the ones who got the girls. I was good at arithmetic and algebra but weak in trigonometry. That didn't matter. I locked in my future career, and the mathematics involved in such a career, starting with calculus, be damned. I wanted to be an astrophysicist, so therefore I deserved to be one. Reality soon hit me between the eyes.

I enrolled in Carleton College in Northfield, Minnesota, with astrophysics in mind. I took Calculus I my first semester and was shocked to discover I didn't understand any of it. I barely passed the class, and only because I memorized everything I could. I knew worse was coming, and finally realized – no astrophysics for me. Sophomore year I declared political science as my major.

Dad chose Carleton and paid the first year's tuition on condition that I spend summers working in the family bookbinding business started by my great-grandfather. Sophomore year I realized I didn't want to be obligated to him anymore, so I demanded he co-sign student loans for me, which he did at Ruth's urging. I now knew I had to get a job to pay for added expenses, so I applied for a job at Gerties' Pizza. Gertie hired me as a weekend delivery guy at $1.35 an hour. I drove an old laundry truck converted for pizza delivery on Friday and Saturday nights and a few evenings during the week. I usually spent Sundays and Mondays studying and drinking.

My daily routine at Carleton was this: Attend classes, hit the books at the library, get to Gerties' about 6 p.m. and return to my dorm room at midnight after several beers. My other jobs during those four years included manning the night desk for the police department and working with a crew that artificially inseminated turkeys (talk about a shitty job). Senior year I clerked in the city's liquor store and bartended at the city's lounge. It came with the ideal perk – as a city employee I could drink for free. I made excellent use of the privilege.

The political science department chairman said I should take every course I could junior year from Reginald D. Lang, the department's political theorist who was retiring in June 1969.

Fall term junior year I took my first class with Lang. The depth and breadth of his knowledge, along with how he taught, excited and intrigued me. I took nine courses from him that year, including several independent studies all focused on theories of politics and history. He helped open my mind and deepened and sharpened my thinking.

Lang was an outcast among the faculty, most of whom were deeply involved in anti-war organizing, which he shunned. I believe he took me under his wing to deepen my knowledge and nurture himself with a promising student who was also bucking the trends of that time. He helped boost my self-confidence and, in my mind, became the affirming male figure I felt I'd never had in my family. And in a way I affirmed him with my rapt attention. But that wasn't the full story.

There was a darker side to this relationship that I uncovered while writing this part of my story. I came to realize that I had secretly relished the fact that Lang was on the outside of things just as I was. I used that to feed my sense of uniqueness and belittle the elite college scene. I also exploited our mentor/pupil relationship with him to cut corners in my work. For example, I undertook several independent studies during the year but I often couldn't meet a deadline because of my drinking and screwing around. I was sly enough to convince him that I was working a lot, so he often gave me a pass. One time he said just to talk about what I had already accomplished and where I was headed in my research. "I think you've done the work, so no need to write it all down," he said and gave me an A+. I believe he and I shared a common need for respect. He was generous because of my admiration for his learning, and I wallowed in his praise for my potential.

I graduated in 1970 and returned home to stay in my old bedroom while waiting for the Selective Service Administration to decide my fate. I had drawn number 214 in the first draft lottery and passed the military physical inspection (I was 1A and eligible to be drafted into the army when I left Carleton). I took tests for military intelligence and was offered an officer's rank if I enlisted. I said no and was thrilled I had when the draft call stopped at 195. So, what now? Graduate school seemed out because I bombed the Graduate Record Exam Advanced Test on Political Science (with Lang, everything was theory, not politics). No more 'Nam threat. I was living at home and didn't have a clue as to what I wanted.

Lang had retired and moved to Evanston, Illinois. We met weekly for lunch, and one day he told me he had sponsored me for a full scholarship to Cambridge University in England. He helped me with the application process, and I was accepted. The day came when I had to decide whether to go or not, and I told Lang that I had decided not to go. I was ashamed, Lang was very disappointed, and we had no further contact.

I just couldn't go. My sense of inferiority was still in full flower. I felt that way at Carleton, and the thought of attending an 800-year-old university with elite students from around the world terrified me. There was no way, I thought, that I could compete on that level.

As bad as I felt about myself, I used that incident to my advantage (or so I thought). For years I'd sit at a bar and tell this Cambridge story to get people to see me not as I was, but as what

I could have been. I told myself that it wasn't my fault that I didn't go to England, it just wasn't the right time. Of course, there never would have been a right time. Looking back, I'm confident that I would have done well at Cambridge, but I'm convinced that had I not sobered up, I would have been nothing more than a condescending, obnoxious, arrogant drunk wearing a black robe and preaching ideas not my own.

Still at home, I needed a job, if no other reason than to get out of the house. I saw an ad in the classifieds for a bartender at a pizza place and was hired full-time. I was a very good bartender and was popular with the regulars. I started drinking, slowly and surreptitiously, every night at about 11:00 to prime myself for closing up and moving to other bars. I usually snuck in the house around 2 a.m., and in the mornings I stayed in bed until Dad and Ruth left for work.

About nine months later, one of the regulars told me of a position with Gallo Winery, which was moving into the Milwaukee market. It was my first job in the liquor business, and my job was to talk liquor retailers into carrying the product line. There were five us, and our boss gathered us every Thursday afternoon to play cards and drink a case or two of Ripple or Boones Farm. It was a drunk-a-thon, pure and simple. I stored my motorcycle in his garage, and one Thursday while very drunk, I rode out on the freeway. I exited a few miles later, rolled to stop light and fell over. Cars honked as I unsteadily righted the bike and rode on. It was a miracle that I didn't crash and burn.

One of my better customers liked my work (a tribute to my father for hammering a solid work ethic into me) and helped me get hired in 1972 by The Christian Brothers winery. I moved to Chicago for a year and then moved to Springfield, Illinois, to work with all of the TCB distributors in downstate Illinois. I covered all of Illinois outside of Chicago to the southern tip at Cairo, which meant I was on the road five or six days a week and given a generous budget to promote the wines and brandy.

My job involved working with salesmen during the day and taking customers and salesmen out to dinner. I of course bought only the Brothers' wine and brandy, and that in quantity—I was an excellent salesman.

Sales substantially increased because I could talk-the-talk and knew the products well, many of them intimately. I loved being on the road, both for the work itself and the sexual flings available in various towns, to say nothing of the nightly opportunity to get drunk on the Brothers' money. I had found the mother lode of perfect setups—I was in my late twenties, recovered quickly from hangovers, tossed sexual affairs aside like bubblegum wrappers, and was well paid for it!

I worked in the liquor industry for seventeen years and ended that career back in Milwaukee with a local liquor bottler. I finally quit the business in June 1989, four years after joining AA and three years after treatment (My counselor in treatment and AA friends had urged me to quit that business, but I was so far in debt that I couldn't risk it).

Those years in the business revealed my steady mental and emotional decline. I drank continuously and lavishly but never during the workday—a key plank in my denial system. My self-confidence faded, and near the end of my liquor career I couldn't make a "cold call" anymore. I was terrified at the thought of going into a new place and making a pitch for my products. I had become a shadow of my former self, full of false bravado, with even less self-confidence. I just couldn't do it anymore.

The end happened during a trip with my boss to Kansas City. We were to meet with the two owners of a large liquor distributor for dinner, and I foolishly agreed to drive us all to the restaurant. The three of them proceeded to get very drunk with business talk regressing to fast cars, fast women, and loud laughter.

I was then four years sober and had no craving to join in; I saw in them what I used to be. I walked to the bathroom mirror and stared into my eyes: "I'm done." Driving back to Milwaukee the following morning, my boss pleaded with me to forgive him – which I did (a bit); but gave him a 30-days' notice anyway. On June 1, 1989, I walked out of the building into fresh air.

CHAPTER 4
MY INTERIOR

*All the Hennessey and weed can't hide, the pain I feel inside,
it's like I'm living just to die.*
--Tupac Shakur

I hide all my fears inside with a "I'm fine."
--Unknown author

Thinking about how I had managed my liquor sales career, I finally realized that on the surface, at least, I fit right in with our culture. As many adults do, I bent to meet its expectations and demands by pursuing financial security at the cost of emotional peace.

To keep up the image that I was fine, never better, I went to work every day except on those mornings when I was too hung over to get out of bed. Every morning I'd leave my apartment – dirty clothes scattered, sink full of dirty dishes, garbage overflowing -- wearing an $800 topcoat, a bright tie, and polished $150 Johnson & Murphy shoes. I looked really good (my most important mask) but felt like hell and knew deep down it was only a charade. I was becoming a ghost haunting myself with no substance.

I dressed well and earned a decent income, but in truth my fancy clothes and top-shelf liquor choices were nothing more than shiny enamel hiding a rotting interior. I held tightly to a distorted view of myself and the world and slouched through every day until 5 p.m. when I could let the dogs run loose.

I'd tell the bartender I was only in for one drink (most of them knew I was in for the night) and eight hours later I'd still be complaining, "I gotta get outta here." But like magic another shot of whatever would appear, and I of course felt honor bound to tip it up and toss it down.

My drinking career was a long descending arc into careless disregard. I grew thoughtless about my life and everyone else's, too. I took greater risks and Death came to sit on my shoulder.

One time I drove with a friend to Carbondale, Illinois, while cuddling Captain Morgan. By the time we arrived I was very drunk and, making a left turn on a busy street, missed running over a guy by an inch. I just laughed at the time, but I could have gotten years, if not life, in the state penitentiary.

I was lucky to have stopped drinking when I did. I hadn't killed anyone yet, even as the odds of doing so were increasing, given how much I was drinking and that I insisted on driving. And I hadn't killed myself yet either. Guns hadn't yet entered my life, but later physical exams when I was in treatment showed that I was only months away from sustaining permanent brain and liver damage.

All that lay ahead. During the last year of my drinking, I seriously thought about buying a gun and blowing my brains out. The idea scared me so much that I chose another way to end my misery—death by drinking. I didn't consciously intend it, because I was too afraid of death to think that thought. My drinking pattern, however, reveals it. I started drinking so much so quickly that even the drunks I hung with were surprised. I would drink a bottle of whatever – scotch, gin, vodka, whisky, anything really – in a matter of a couple hours, with shots of schnapps to sweeten the way. "What the hell's the matter with you," they'd ask. "Are you crazy?"

Yes, I was. I was losing my mind.

About a year before I quit, I started drinking alone at home, something I had never done before. I was always a downtown, fancy joint drinker – shot and beer joints were for losers, not me. I was the guy who, in a busy nightclub, tipped the waitress $20 the first time and said, "Forget about everyone else in here, pay attention to my glass and this table, and you'll make a lot of money. When this glass is half empty, fill it."

I had become careless with my life and the lives of others, too. I refused protected sex because I didn't care about my partner's health. I ate less, slept little, and drank more. I married a woman I was in lust with, cheated on her within thirty days of tying what I considered a slip knot, and filed for divorce in five months. I wiped people out of my life for not giving me the attention and affirmation I demanded. Their names make for a long list.

The final act of my drinking began in September 1985.
As a kid I had loved books, sports, camping--everything outdoors. By age thirty-seven, having drunk enough booze to float a good-sized boat, my mind started to slip away. I stopped reading, watching the news, having sex, or going on walks. My daily life had become trashy and shallow. I feared the future, wallowed in the past, and hated the present. I had become a turtle, pulling my head back into my shell at the merest whiff of danger. Near the end, I locked myself inside, eyes closed to the world, waiting.

I became deeply depressed. Booze no longer worked its magic by infusing some excitement in my daily life. At night I started drinking alone for the first time. I'd pull the curtains closed with only one light on, sit in my chair with a large glass of booze and a towel to soak up tears. I was spiraling down to meet a pine box six feet underground.

CHAPTER 5
YES, MIRACLES DO HAPPEN

This was the day my Earth stood still
(with a nod to the movie)

By the time September 1985 rolled around, I was a basket case. I still found some relief in drinking, but the good times were gone, and I was drowning. My life had withered to working a day liquor salesman job I hated, bartending four or five times a week, and heavy drinking every night.

I had essentially become comatose. Reading books and newspapers, going to the movies, hiking in the woods, or engaging in sex were all washed away in a flood of alcohol. I hung out with my drunk buddies for the sole purpose of drinking more. It was all I had left.

And then…

It was a late Friday night. I was tending bar at a hip nightclub in downtown Milwaukee when a waitress told me I had a phone call—it was Nancy.

About ten years before, Nancy had worked in a restaurant I managed, and I lusted after her. She seemed to be blessed with an earthy understanding of life and always talked about what could be for her. I didn't get what she was talking about, and she probably sensed that in me. We didn't connect then because she was heading to Colorado; she offered no guarantees, and I flinched at the thought of uncertain change. But out of the blue, here she was, all these years later, calling me on a Friday night.

"Bob, I want you to come out to Colorado and help me celebrate my thirty-fifth birthday," she said.

I was shocked to hear her voice, and knee jerked my natural response: "Probably not." I told her I would call the next day.

She talked me into making the trip. I stepped off the plane in Denver, and there she stood with her two kids. We drove north outside Longmont and up into the foothills along a winding forest road and parked at her cabin.

There I stood, an emotional wreck looking to be saved from myself, and there she was, as beautiful as I remembered and living in a cabin in the Rocky Mountain foothills! It was my dream come true, and I instantly fell in … "love" isn't the right word, because I now know I saw her as a life jacket that would float me out of the life I knew, the woman who would take care of me. She would do for me what I couldn't, or wouldn't, do for myself.

I swooned at this vision of love in the foothills, and of course I was hallucinating. Nevertheless, for the first time in a long time I laughed a lot and enjoyed myself. We of course drank like fish and had sex, and I flew back to Milwaukee on the pinkest of clouds.

For the next several weeks I schemed how I could find a way to be with her. It wasn't going to be easy. I owned three duplex houses, which I had bought a year before I quit, with the thought that my life would get better if I owned some real estate. I financed them with a crazy nineteen percent interest funding scheme I thought was genius because no one had ever tried it before. There was a good reason for that – it was stupid scheme which guaranteed that I would end up in serious debt.

To get free of those properties, I decided to drop off the key at the financing company, sneak away from other financial responsibilities, and drive straight along Interstate 80 to her cabin. I fantasized her rushing to hug and kiss me while her kids screamed and scampered in delight. That balloon was about to pop.

The last drink I remember taking was early morning on November 2, 1985, at about 4:00 a.m. I had tended bar Friday night until closing at 2:00 a.m., and with others went down the alley to another joint and continued drinking at a fast pace while playing bar dice. It was a fast game with the loser of each round buying shots of whatever sat on the back bar. With four of us rolling, each game would last about ten minutes, after which another shot of booze went down my throat chased with a scotch and water. We'd pound that dice cup for an hour or more.

That last shot was Green Chartreuse, an herbal French liqueur. I can still see that green glass moving toward my lips, when blink! Everything goes dark, just like every other blackout I don't remember. My cronies later told me I drank for another couple hours.

Apparently, I drove home, unlocked my front door, and fell into bed, but I don't remember any of it. I woke up Sunday morning still fully clothed, so sick with nausea and headache I couldn't get up at first but prayed to the flush god all day. I stayed in bed with a terrible hangover.

The next day, Monday, I went to work and wore sunglasses to hide my bloodshot eyes. The only food I could keep down was chocolate milk.

Tuesday morning, I felt better. Today's the day, I thought, to tell Nancy that I'd soon be on my way. At 10:45 a.m., I stopped at 92nd and Capital Drive in Milwaukee and plunked quarters into the pay phone in front of a large liquor store, one of my customers.

Nancy answered and as I excitedly told her my plan, she broke in: "What's the matter with you? Are you out of your fucking mind?"

And then it happened. *The Miracle* . . .

Suddenly, shockingly, I knew I had to quit drinking. That thought came out of nowhere. It was a conscious thought I'd never had before, and it exploded in my head. I almost passed out. I was so stunned I hung up on Nancy (she was still ranting) and sat back down in my car. "I have to quit drinking" engulfed my mind.

I could see clearly that I had to quit – not why, just that I needed to. How to describe that moment, or make sense of it? A meteor strike? A two-by-four upside the head?

How to explain it? I'm not religious, but I believe to this day it was a miracle which saved me from drinking myself to death. Maybe my guardian angel finally got fed up, grabbed me by the scruff of my neck, and threw me through the door of AA with the commandment, "Go to work!" Or perhaps the universe responded to all the bad vibes I had sent out by boomeranging my brain with some good stuff. Whatever it was, my life shifted in an instant. I didn't realize that I had been shoved to the cusp of a great psychic upheaval.

My mind reeling, I felt desperate to see Ron, a customer of mine on my liquor route that day. About an hour later I sat on his rundown couch, my head in my hands.

He got off the phone: "What's happened to you? You look like you've seen a ghost."

"I don't know what happened," I said. "All I know is I have to stop drinking."

Ron stared at me over the top of his glasses for several moments. "You know, all these years you've asked me to go out for a few drinks, and I always said no," he said. He always told me that "one is too many, and a thousand ain't enough," which of course I didn't get at all. "But now maybe you're ready to hear this: I'm a member of AA, and you're not leaving this room until we've talked."

Talk about another miracle! I don't remember his words, but I can guess. They're the same ones I say to newcomers: "You've been on a very dark road, but you don't have to drink anymore. I've been there, and I guarantee you that sobriety will give you a totally different, free and happy life."

He let me go only after I had agreed to meet him that evening for a cup of coffee at the Twelve Step Club, which was an easy walk from my house. Looking back, it all just seemed to fall into place – first the gong of a celestial bell, then a friend's intervention, and finally an AA club in my neighborhood.

I asked Ron to be my sponsor, and he told me repeatedly to "Hang in there, wait for the magic to happen." Which I did, and it did.

I was also blessed by being immediately relieved of the compulsion to drink. I've been to numerous funerals of those who took their lives because the cravings never stopped. But my default position of calling all rules "bullshit" almost took me out the door. But I stuck it out. Over the years I've known many in AA who also hung in there and now also live abundant, joyous, robust lives with new life tapestries woven in faith, hope, happiness and trust.

***

I'll be talking more now about the 12 Steps and 12 Traditions, so I've listed them here for those who aren't familiar with them. I talk more extensively of my experience with the Steps in Chapter 9. Other 12-Step programs, including Narcotics Anonymous, cast these Steps and Traditions in their own words.

An important thing to note: These Steps mention alcohol only two times, which to me has always meant that addiction recovery is a process of detoxing the mind, and these Steps are the pathway to spiritual healing.

The Twelve Steps
1: We admitted we were powerless over alcohol -- that our lives had become unmanageable.
2: Came to believe that a Power greater than ourselves could restore us to sanity.

3: Made a decision to turn our will and our lives over to the care of God as we understood Him.

4: Made a searching and fearless moral inventory of ourselves.

5: Admitted to God, to ourselves and to another human being the exact nature of our wrongs.

6: Were entirely ready to have God remove all these defects of character.

7: Humbly asked Him to remove our shortcomings.

8: Made a list of all persons we had harmed and became willing to make amends to them all.

9: Made direct amends to such people wherever possible, except when to do so would injure them or others.

10: Continued to take personal inventory, and when we were wrong promptly admitted it.

11: Sought through prayer and meditation to improve our conscious contact with God, as we understood Him, praying only for knowledge of His will for us and the power to carry that out.

12: Having had a spiritual awakening as the result of these Steps, we tried to carry this message to alcoholics and to practice these principles in all our affairs.

The Twelve Traditions

1: Our common welfare should come first; personal recovery depends on AA unity.

2: For our group purpose there is but one ultimate authority – a loving God as he may express Himself in our group conscience. Our leaders are but trusted servants; they do not govern.

3: The only requirement for AA membership is a desire to stop drinking.

4: Each group should be autonomous, except in matters affecting other groups or AA as a whole.

5: Each group has but one primary purpose: to carry its message *to the alcoholic who still suffers.*

6: An AA group ought never endorse, finance, or lend the AA name to any related facility or outside enterprise, lest problems of money, property, and prestige divert us from our primary purpose.

7: Every AA group ought to be fully self-supporting, declining outside contributions.

8: Alcoholics Anonymous should remain forever non-professional, but our service centers may employ special workers.

9: AA, as such, ought never be organized; but we may create service boards or committees directly responsible to those they serve.

10: Alcoholics Anonymous has no opinion on outside issues; hence the AA name ought never be drawn into public controversy.

11: Our public relations policy is based on attraction rather than promotion; we need always maintain personal anonymity at the level of press, radio, and films.

12: Anonymity is the spiritual foundation of all our traditions, ever reminding us to place principles above personalities.

CHAPTER 6
AA TO MY RESCUE

*The first step towards getting somewhere is to decide that
you're not going to stay where you are.*
(Unknown author)

*You cannot swim for new horizons until you have courage
to lose sight of the shore.*
--William Faulkner

I attended my very first meeting that same night. I find it hard
to describe what I felt entering the Great Unknown in that hour.
Fear? Confusion? Shame? Yes, to those feelings and many more.

The Twelve Step Club was home to a wide variety of folks
from an assortment of backgrounds (It's still going strong with recovery programs for alcoholics, drug abusers, opioid abusers and
more). I met many like me, raised in upper-middle-class homes,
sitting across from others who had grown up in poverty and home-
lessness.

Blacks, whites, and Latinos, men and women, walked through
its door. Many members had distinguished careers in medicine
and engineering; others held advanced college degrees. Some had
received little quality education and grew up in neighborhoods
with few job opportunities. Quite a few were homeless. That place
hosted a broad mix of folks of all colors and backgrounds, but
once inside, all of us were addicts and therefore equal. There is no
caste system in AA.

AA is the great leveler, its only purpose to help one another
stay sober. I watched amazed as a homeless Black man huddled
with a wealthy white man new to the rooms, both of them sipping

coffee and talking about sobriety. The Club was an amazing place, where color and status meant absolutely nothing. Such a place was way outside my tight little white-world envelope, but I grew to love it. Why? Because AA saved my life.

The Club had repurposed an old neighborhood corner grocery store. You walked into a large room with about a dozen tables with a coffee bar in one corner and a rack of candy bars. Large posters laying out the 12 Steps and 12 Traditions hung on a wall surrounded by inspirational sayings: Easy Does It, One Day at a Time, Keep it Simple Stupid. Meetings were held upstairs in the old apartment rooms.

I walked in early and saw about twenty men and women sitting around tables holding coffee mugs talking and laughing. Some looked me over, as if to say, "Who's the new guy?" I panicked and walked over to get some coffee. For about ten minutes, I stood facing away from the room in a corner and read notices as if I was serious. I didn't turn around because I just knew everyone was looking at me. I was scared shitless. Then Ron finally walked in and rescued me. He took me in hand to meet some of the old timers playing cards and drinking coffee.

One guy stood up and got in my face: "How are you and God?"

"Fuck God," I said.

Ron ushered me away to the 12-Steps and 12-Traditions hangings. "Read these, this is how it works," he said.

I read "Fearless moral inventory." "Humbly… spiritual awakening." It could have been written in Sanskrit for all I understood about such concepts. I kind of growled at "Turn our will and our lives over to the care of God…" Bullshit, I thought.

In the meeting, I was introduced as a newcomer, and as is customary, everyone talked about the First Step and their experience, strength, and hope in finding sobriety. I don't remember anything that was said (but I can guess), and at the end of the meeting we all stood and held hands for the Lord's Prayer. "What the hell kind of place is this?" I thought.

However, I saw real happiness in the eyes of some around that table. Since I didn't have it, I was acutely aware of others who did. And they seemed to be better people than me. I recall the book, Zen and the Art of Motorcycle Maintenance, by Robert M. Pirsig and his discussion of quality: you know it when you see it.

I had always wanted more than anything to feel happy, and in my teen years, booze provided some of that by dulling my terrors and anger. I loved the "off my rocker" feel of it more than the taste, and just the act of drinking and the anticipation of getting drunk excited me. Alcohol never brought me any real happiness or a deep sense of well-being. Something always seemed to be missing which I couldn't find, so I held on to the only thing I knew for sure -- a bottle.

Suddenly I realized that I was with happy people, and I wanted what they had. I wanted it so much that I came back the next evening to be with them and kept coming to meetings. I attended meetings like clockwork: every weekday evening and sometimes twice on weekends. Just being around people made me feel better, and the stories I listened to showed me the way to go.

I knew I had to quit drinking, but I didn't think I was an alcoholic. I listened to others share their stories of drinking or drug use. Most of their stories confirmed my own denial. One guy, for example, talked about waking up from a blackout in a gunfight with the Tennessee State Patrol. Another said police caught him breaking into a house to steal a stereo to fence for cash to buy more drugs. Many talked about the choice given by judges: AA or jail.

"If *that's* being an alcoholic, then I'm not one because I never did stuff like that," I told myself.

I leaned back in the chair, with a smug look on my face, thinking maybe I wasn't worth much, but I was a damn site better than these losers. I believed I was the most honest guy around – I never stole anything, made sure to tip waitresses well, and always returned the correct change. Judges and jails never knew my name. I had never wrecked a car or run anyone over (I got close a couple of times; often driving in black outs and waking up not knowing the condition of my car's front bumper).

At first, I couldn't admit the lies I told to myself and others – that came later with hard work. How I had cheated my employer by not working as best I could; how I had cheated on my first wife shortly after we married (see Step Four in Part II). How I had betrayed friends with oaths of love and loyalty I never intended and buried my deepest feelings. How my distorted view of Dad and Don warped my relationship with my family... the list goes on. I was a tortured, amoral, emotional wreck. I looked good on the outside but was always lonely, even in a crowd. I had become an ephemera drifting on the edge of things.

Eventually I met two 12 Step Club members who saved me from walking out the door. Tom and Nona took me under their wing and became my friends. Tom, a fiftyish Irish drunk, had a sharp and truthful tongue that often called out my bullshit. One evening I told him I was thinking of buying a motorcycle and riding into the sunset.

"You'll be drunk before you hit the state line," Tom said. "You're really fucked up, and you better get your ass in treatment. Tom was finishing his thirty days at The McBride Center for the Impaired Professional. "You better get in there, or you'll get drunk."

Nona was a Black woman with a dozen years of sobriety. She shared her own stories and encouraged me to stay calm and expect the best. Her tongue was sharp when I needed it to be, and she never sacrificed a word. She pushed me to consider treatment.

"Once the booze is out of your system, you'll feel so much better, so hang in there," she often said.

Tom and Nona shared their secrets, which gave me the courage to start exhuming my own. They lifted me when I was down, taught me how to laugh and be happy again, and treated me as an equal. Here is some of what I learned from them:

I needed to hang out with folks who were serious about recovery and not just goof around. It took me some time to feel comfortable around others, but I know the special folks sitting around those tables and drinking coffee really kept me from going back out. Without Tom and Nona, I'm not sure I would have stayed sober.

My sole purpose was to heal myself and not someone else. I learned that hard lesson early by trying to sponsor other men when I was so obviously adrift in my own flaws. I had to do my own work and accept that I'm not God. But I admit I struggled with giving up the throne.

Pay attention to HALT, or Hungry, Angry, Lonely, Tired. This acronym, posted on every AA meeting wall, is crucial for sober living, and its importance never fades. I can feel when I'm stretching my limits and not taking care of myself – I turn judgmental and dissatisfied with things, and generally settle into a crappy mood. Eight months after my last drink, I decided to follow their advice and checked into the McBride Center.

CHAPTER 7
TRUTH HITS HOME

There are years that ask questions and years that answer.
--Zora Neale Hurston, folklorist and author

Faith is the bird that feels the light when the dawn is still dark.
--Rabindranath Tagore, Bengali poet and musician

I was emotionally stuck and knew it. Something wasn't right and I felt it.

Some things had changed – I accepted that I was an alcoholic and had done some stupid things. But I stayed a rock on the recovery shore pushing against the tide of recovery lessons I was afraid to learn.

Everything seemed fine – I felt good physically, I went to work every day to the job I hated and banked my paychecks. I wasn't craving alcohol, even though I had occasional drinking dreams that scared me. In one dream I took a drink in despair and cried. But I didn't feel right. Something was out of whack, but I didn't know what.

What I really wanted was a break, a vacation away from it all.

Tom and Nona told me to get my butt in treatment, but I wallowed in the admiration of those who found out I was the odd guy who was staying sober on his own, and I wasn't ready to let that go. I thought I was better than them, and to prove it I memorized key passages in the Big Book so I could give the right answers. I read six reflection books every morning instead of the mere two most others thought adequate. Tom and Nona saw right through me and, at times at a loss for words, they just shook their heads.

I still wanted a break. One morning I looked at my company

insurance policy and discovered it would cover thirty days of in-patient chemical dependency treatment. That was gold-plate insurance back then and a rarity today. Gee, I thought, I could go into treatment, have a vacation from work... and relax! So, I took Tom's advice and scheduled my intake.

I told my bosses when I quit drinking and they were all very supportive. I now went to the company owner and told him I thought I needed to go into treatment, that I just wasn't feeling right, and he told me I should do whatever I needed for myself. That was extremely generous of him, but I wasn't being honest, and I knew it. I told him ten days would probably be enough time because I was past the need for a detox.

What in fact I did need and was still totally unaware of was a detox of my thinking. That was soon to come.

I had no idea what was waiting for me at McBride even after Tom's colorful stories about his own experiences there. Piece of cake, I thought, and in that spirit, I bought new clothes intending to hit on women and I took a racket and balls figuring I'd have time for tennis.

Here I want to interject by comparing sobriety with emotional sobriety. I was eight months sober and didn't want to drink ever again, and physically felt much better. That was sobriety for me. I was about to discover a much deeper and darker pit inside me that I had no clue existed. Entering treatment was my first step along the path to emotional sobriety. To earn that I had to move inside with honesty and self-responsibility to confront my past, and with tears, wash away the lies and bullshit.

On a Friday afternoon in July 1986, McBride welcomed me in through a steel door that slammed shut and was locked. Attendants emptied my bag, checked all my clothes, uncapped my toothpaste tube, and disassembled my digital alarm clock. What the hell is this place? I wondered.

I was led to my room, unpacked, and then moseyed into the community room. I sat next to Joe, a friend I had met at meetings. As always to quiet my uneasiness I told jokes, many of them raunchy bar jokes because that's all I knew. I started feeling comfortable until a counselor walked in and barked: "What is this, Joe's tap?" He stared hard at me, and my stomach clenched.

Later that afternoon, we were called into a large circle – about thirty of us – to watch the counselors tear into a woman who refused to go to meetings. "I'm not a drunk, I'm only here because my husband made me," she said. They kicked her out that evening. I knew then that I was in deep shit. I soon discovered how deep.

Our daily schedule included meetings in small groups with our counselor and one of the doctors running the McBride Center. My group included about ten others and Dean, our counselor, who led the questions and discussion. The doctor usually sat quietly and took notes.

I was the new guy, so they let me sit on the sideline for three or four days until Dean and his icy blue eyes turned to me: "Bob, why don't you tell us about your drinking." I felt like a panicked deer in headlights – my brain froze and didn't know what to say. Dean excused himself to go to the bathroom. I squeezed a few words out; that I had started drinking when I was twelve, worked as a sales representative in the liquor industry and tended bar on the side, blah, blah, blah. I sat back feeling satisfied at the good job I'd made of it. I thought I had passed the test until Dean walked back into the room.

He looked at his watch, looked me in the eyes, and said, "You summarized your twenty-five years of drinking in five minutes." A moment passed. "When are you going to cut the bullshit and get honest about your drinking?"

Yikes! I was in deep shit.

I accepted that I was an alcoholic but didn't yet understand how drinking had affected my life and how my behavior hurt others. I believed I was a high-class exception to all the others who were so obviously just drunks or coke heads, because I never did any of the shocking things or suffered the physical and mental damage they experienced (I was to learn how close I came). Some stories were so bizarre I thought they were lies. My story was of a higher caliber, I thought.

I didn't like who I was, hated my job and feared the future—but hey, I wasn't like them. I was better than them. I was cheating my employer, but so what? I betrayed my wife, but she caused me to do it. I was an asshole, but I had earned the right to be one. My bottom line -- I deserved a break.

In fact, the break I got was in my mind and heart.

I left that group scared and badly shaken. Suddenly things seemed less sure, and I felt like I was sliding downhill. I realized I needed to take this program seriously. I stopped joking around and seriously thought about my drinking. That shift happened at a good time -- our next assignment was to write an autobiography, a story of my life so far, as a prelude to tackling the Fourth Step.

My first thought was, this'll be easy as pie. All I had to do was blame my drinking on everyone else. All I had to do was write down all the stories I had been telling myself for twenty-five years; that Dad was a bastard who didn't love me, Mom's dying had screwed me up, and it was the world's unfairness that made my life miserable. Women didn't like me or wanted too much, and I was the best kind of guy because I was honest about giving back the right change, and on and on.

It was a testament to my innocence of any wrongdoing, and a declaration that my life was shit but that wasn't my fault. I knocked out over twenty pages and believed I had aced the test. I wrote all of it like I read The Big Book in my early days – so I could be sure to answer any question and fill in the blanks to be just fine. (The official AA text is "Alcoholics Anonymous," commonly referred to by members as "The Big Book.")

Each of us had our own room. Mine wasn't very big but it had a single bed, a small closet, a bathroom with a shower, and a desk. A couple nights later I tossed and turned because something felt off. I got up and stood at the desk looking down on those pages, and I knew, in a flash of insight, that what I had written was bullshit. It cracked my shield so I could see some truth of what drinking had cost me and what I had done to others. I cried for the first time in years, and my tears kept coming. I tore up those pages and started over.

For days I cried all the time. I cried in the shower, I cried rewriting my autobiography, I cried trying to be honest, I cried at finally beginning to see my part in everything that happened to me. I wasn't sure what it all meant, but it felt like my guts had been ripped open. It was the first time I had felt any responsibility for my life. My inner vision was still really limited, but I could see a tiny light at the end of a long dark tunnel.

Writing all that down was painful and felt shameful, but it confirmed what I'd always believed: I was a fraud and a failure. I began whipping myself for being the worst person in the world, no one was as bad as me, etc. etc.

Each of us had to read our bios to the group. At my turn I read the first sentence and broke down in tears. Dean said we'd try again tomorrow. The next day, I couldn't get any words out over my tears and sobs. The doctor said tomorrow might be the day.

The next day, I finally read my world-shattering bio out loud, with tears and a shaky voice adding some punctuation. To my surprise, no one seemed shocked. What, no one believed me? I listened to others read their stories and began to understand that I was a fellow traveler with everyone else, that I was no longer alone or unique in my pain and despair. My life was a medley like theirs, differing only in the score. Understanding that, and feeling relief, was a first compass point, a first true directional bearing in my recovery toward real sobriety.

It also proved to be the first tiny awareness that I was an individual in and of myself, a real person no longer a creation of somebody else's definition. That insight created my first understanding of and empathy for others. It lifted a huge burden from my heart, as I no longer had to hide in fear of being found out. I could start breathing my own air.

I carried so much inner baggage. Treatment led me to a place I needed most – honesty, about who I was, responsibility for my role in creating the life I had been living, and a sense of well-being and happiness. I wasn't yet joyous or free of my demons, but I was aware of their chains and knew a way to break them. I just needed the courage. And a lot of humility.

I had to calculate how much money I had blown on alcohol. I came up with $180,000, which in 2020 dollars is an astonishing $439K (and probably more than $500K if I had invested it all). That number represents only what I personally spent – a lot more floated my way. I had access to free booze while bartending, expense accounts for promoting the alcohol brands I sold, and many freebies from bartenders at my favorite joints. Yes indeed, I drank a lot.

Our next task was to write a formal Fourth Step with Dean at our side, and follow that with a Fifth Step to share our story with a chaplain.

My memory of the rest of the time has faded, but I do remember not wanting to leave when the thirty days were up. I didn't want to go back to my liquor sales job – the counselors didn't want me to, either – or back home to the large empty house. I had bonded with several people in treatment, Joe in particular, and wanted to stay in the womb. The center was my new comfort zone. But the world waited, and my insurance ended.

During my exit interview with my doctor, I discovered just how out of touch with my body I had become. . He asked me if I noticed any changes in my body, and I said, "Yes, I'm having bowel movements every day!"

"How often did you have those when you were drinking," he asked.

"Maybe once or twice a week," I said.

"You have to remember you're eating three meals a day now, so your body functions differently," he said.

"Oh."

I noticed other changes. My lower lip, split open and bleeding for years due to chronic dehydration despite boatloads of scotch and water, had healed. I had gained some weight, the light blotches on face had disappeared, and I bought glasses so I could see road signs and center lines.

I was discharged on a Friday afternoon and drove home to the house I had bought in early October 1985, about a month before I quit drinking. Irony of ironies, I never had a drink in that place, even though I had been drinking alone in my old apartment.

My new place was 1920s beautiful. It had leaded glass windows, maple and oak floors, and molded plaster ceilings. There was a full basement, two large apartments with maids' quarters on the third floor. The house greeted me with silence. I started to feel my old uneasiness in the looming dusk.

Rattling around that large house, I immediately fell back into old patterns – isolating, haunting night fears, simmering orneriness. I went to work every day with a dark cloud above my head, but I walked to AA meetings every evening to find the fun, laughter, and comfort with Tom and Nona I craved.

I always felt amazed at how alike we were, and how at ease I felt with the men and women I knew in AA. On most nights after the meetings were over and the coffee urns had run dry, people started to head home, but I hated to leave. Then the walk home into a lonely, dimly lit house.

There was a moment when I almost relapsed. In a phone call, my Dad said something to me (I don't remember what exactly) and I slammed down the phone. I was so angry that I rushed out and bought a half-gallon of ice cream and rented some porn tapes. I got back home and shoveled in ice cream while jerking off to those tapes. I was teetering on the knife's edge -- another push from anyone from anywhere could have sent me out to a bar or a bottle.

The next morning, I woke up feeling hung over from anger and sugar. I was ashamed, even scared at how I had acted but still angry at Dad. But then, as would so often happen to me, another epiphany bloomed -- I knew I couldn't live alone anymore. I needed to live with others to stop isolating. I knew that if I continued to live alone and apart, I'd probably slither back to drinking.

I was lucky. I met two guys at a Tuesday evening meeting at McBride who were desperate. They were both about to leave the half-way house but didn't feel ready to go home and deal with their angry families. So, I invited them to move in with me. Like magic, the instant they walked in the door, I felt comfortable, safe, and open. I no longer felt isolated and alone. We'd sit around a table, drink coffee, and talk about recovery. My emotional sobriety took hold then and my inner work truly began.

CHAPTER 8
ME AND MY FAMILY

All happy families are alike: each unhappy family is
unhappy in its own way.
--Leo Tolstoy

Love me or hate me, both are in my favor.
If you love me, I will always be in your heart, and if you hate me,
I will always be in your mind.
--Qandeel Baloch, Pakistani model and actress

Was I born an alcoholic? Almost certainly. But that's only one key to what happened to me. Catastrophe was another.

Before I go into that, here's a look at my family.

I was born into a family that by appearance alone could have modeled for a Norman Rockwell painting – white, upper-middle class with two parents smiling at three wholesome-looking kids. We kids were born in the 1940s, and our parents, Norman and Elaine, were born in the post-World War I era. The social norms my parents inherited from their parents – display outward success as proof of worth and carry on in the face of trouble -- molded all of us by the cultural expectations of the white, above-average family with an above-average income living in an above-average house on an above-average street.

Don, Peg, and I were above average students earning good grades, and we never got involved in below-average behavior, beyond typical childhood pranks (I used to swipe Hostess Twinkies from a small store on the way to elementary school and I tossed wet leaves in open car windows on Trick-or-Treat nights). I followed my brother and sister through the same elementary, junior high, and high schools, often with the same teachers. A usual refrain I came to hate: "Oh, you're Don's and Peg's brother, well I hope you're as good a student as they were." If my grades and behavior wasn't as good as theirs, I heard about it at home.

Ours was a classic 1950s family. Dad ran the family bookbinding business, and Mom ran the household. She did all the cooking, laundry, house cleaning, and daily discipline of her rambunctious children. Dad's household work was outside – no dishwashing for him, and the only cooking he ever did was on a barbecue grill. He kept our Buick spotless, the house in no-peeling-paint condition and windows gleaming; weeded the rose gardens and dusted for mites; and fed the lawn, a dark Kentucky Bluegrass green, multiple doses of fertilizer.

We attended a conservative Lutheran Church in which John Calvin might have felt at home. My father believed, and continually reminded me, that we manifest our salvation through good works, solid behavior, and worldly success. "We must pay rent through good works for our space on Earth," he always said. By that he meant that work in and of itself was a moral virtue brooking no exception for any of the seven deadly sins. "Work makes life sweet," and "Patience is a virtue," were other favorites he hoped I would absorb. I can honestly say they soaked in, but I balked at every chance to live them.

Dad was emotionally abused by his mother, Norma, who, I believe, suffered mental and emotional trauma as a child. His father, Gallus, seemed to love fishing and mischief more than he loved his son. Dad was the only child of what seemed to be a dysfunctional marriage, and to prove his worth to them and the world, Dad became the straightest of straight shooters. He could be as surprisingly warm-hearted in giving his time and energy to help others and as he was severely judgmental and strict. He held himself to his own standards. By appearance he was on the short side, a bit overweight with a knife-edged flat top haircut and always well-dressed. He walked with head thrust forward as if marching toward righteousness.

As befitted his strict standard that everyone should be equally treated, Dad imposed on me the same rules he had developed for Don and Peg, who were six and four years older than me respectively. I know now that Dad's goal was to treat each of us kids the same, leaving me, the youngest, at the end of the line, shackled to the same bedtimes, clothing styles, haircuts, house chores, etc. But even as a small kid, and certainly in my teens, I believed my father's pride in my older brother's accomplishments placed me in a minor orbit in the family constellation.

Now I fully understand the reason why. After Don survived polio and came home from the hospital, Dad and Mom hovered over him to protect him from harm. I sensed the change in the focus of their attention and, and being only seven years old, didn't understand what that meant. Instead, I took it to mean that I suddenly meant less to them than I used to, that I was consigned to a lower order, and made me angry. Not only at Dad, but Don, too.

Hoping to draw his attention, I tried to be like my Dad in certain ways – judgmental and hardworking. I tried to outdo Don in my juvenile way by acting up, but that only drew put-downs from my parents, which affirmed my sense of being the family Ishmael. I felt that way for years. Don went on to a successful college career and a prominent job in the chemical industry which Dad loved to brag about to friends and family. Don's success was a ball and chain I'd have to drag along no matter what I did. I saw no way past that, but one day I tried to hit Dad's funny bone.

Our front lawn was Dad's testament to our family's character. You'd turn the corner onto our street and think God Almighty Himself had blessed our lawn. I chuckle to think that our patch of green could have been seen from space. Caring for the lawn was a rite unto itself with set rules for the mowing, trimming, and cultivating. I followed those rules religiously, cutting the grass in a north/south, east/west grid. But one day, when I was about eleven, I had an impish thought: I'll mow it just like those groundskeepers do with the Braves' outfield at County Stadium—diagonally. I was thrilled with the results. Dad, less so. "What the hell did you do to the lawn?" he yelled, and ordered me to re-mow it The Right Way.

Through my first three years on this planet, my sister Peg doted on me so much that I had yet to speak a word. I had no reason to, because she fetched whatever I pointed at. Dad was so concerned about my not talking that he asked the family pediatrician to make a house call. The doctor watched as Peg chased to and fro and said, "You keep her away from him, and he'll talk." Dad told me I spoke a few days later at dinner to everyone's surprise: "Pass the salt and pepper please."

The lesson I learned from that coddling was that I deserved to have someone else take care of my needs, which of course kicked open the door to blame and resentment when people didn't do what I thought they should. This pattern echoes in me even now, especially around service I believe I deserve at restaurants and big box stores. I'm working on it.

Don and I lived in different worlds when I was a kid because he was six years older. It's no wonder we did little together; he played sports while I played in my sandbox. I was in grade school when he was dating in high school. His hormones raged while mine still slept.

The family myth shattered with the death of my mother. I look at my parents' wedding picture and see a tall, lithe, beautiful young woman with long, flowing hair standing with Dad, a bit rigid in posture, with a happy but controlled smile. She was the love of his life, and she died of cancer at age forty-one. A large part of me died with her. (See Note 6 on grief.)

The cataclysm of Mom's death broke my heart, gutted my faith, and obliterated most of my memories of her. I do remember her reading to me as I snuggled in bed, and scrubbing the dirt from my ears. But I can barely recall her image without looking at pictures. I've watched old 16-mm films from when I was a toddler showing her in motion, laughing and smiling as I wriggled in her lap. The films give her movement and life I don't remember.

Praying for a miracle and trying to protect us, Dad kept secret just how sick with cancer she was. She was in and out of the hospital for two years, and whenever I asked about her, Dad said not to worry. Just pray and all will be okay, I remember him telling me.

Her unexpected death was a shattering psychic upheaval that changed all our lives. Don, Peg, and I shared a deep guilt. How could we not, when for two summers, while Mom suffered in a hospital, we spent every kid's dream of fishing, water skiing, and listening to 1950s rock n' roll to our hearts' content at my Grandmother Schober's cottage on Lac la Belle outside of Oconomowoc, Wisconsin. We could do pretty much what we wanted outside the cottage, because grandma ignored us as long as we obeyed her rules. Dad came to the lake every Sunday on his way back to Milwaukee after visiting Mom in a hospital in Madison.

I remember belly-flopping contests off the end of the pier with my friend Lenny, playing croquet with Don and Peg's friends, and volleying tennis balls with my great-aunt Flora. We didn't have a care in the world those two summers, assured by Dad that everything would be okay. Finally, her doctors admitted they couldn't do anything more for her and told her to go home and spend what time she had left with her kids.

Dad brought her to the lake on a Saturday in August 1958. I barely recognized her at first, her face gaunt from pain and her body shriveled from the cancer eating her alive. Then she tried to smile at me. I was shocked. I think I backed away from her.

But Dad had a business to run, so he drove home to Milwaukee while Mom stayed at the lake with us for about two weeks. The only bed for her was inside the cottage, where she lay bedridden most days. We three kids took turns feeding her in bed when she was too weak to get up.

One day at noon as we sat around grandma's kitchen table for lunch, Mom suddenly shuffled into the kitchen. In great pain, she marshalled all the strength she had left to keep a smile on her face and walk unaided from her bedroom across the kitchen floor to join us at the table. I remember sitting there absolutely stunned, watching her struggle to stay on her feet. I think she sat down with us, but I don't remember.

When school was about to start, Dad drove us home and put Mom back in the hospital.

On September 18, 1958, Dad came home and gathered us kids and my grandmother in the sunroom. I remember Peg and I sat on the floor, Don sat in the recliner, and grandma on the couch. Dad sat across from us at the old telephone desk and told us: "Your mother died this afternoon." He picked up the phone and started dialing to give family friends the news.

Don cried, Peg screamed, I exploded. Furious, I rushed into the kitchen and started throwing things at a wall. I could hear Dad talking on the phone, not to us. Grandma followed me into the kitchen and barked, "Stop that!" There was no talking, no comforting, no nothing. Peg went to her room and slammed the door. I don't remember what Don did or what I did next.

Dad was so crushed by Mom's death he didn't know what to do or how to handle it. He couldn't, and wouldn't, talk with us about her and what her death meant. He even went so far as to forbid us from talking with our friends' parents about her death. I now realize he only wanted to help us and figured that keeping up appearances would dull our pain.

We were supposed to still look good, behave well, study hard and act like nothing had happened. My brother and I carried on with our chores; my sister was given the job of cooking all the meals and cleaning. Dad sat at the head of the table with Mom's empty chair on his right, which I couldn't avoid looking at.

Dad had no choice but to keep moving ahead, because the business called out its demands each day. But he also needed to be married, felt the need for a wife for love. He met Ruth on a trip to New York City through a mutual friend.

Ruth married into our family a year later. That news also came as a surprise announcement from Dad and caused some upset. Ruth was a brave woman to marry into a family of needy, angry kids with a mother-in-law intent on criticizing her at every chance. Dad and Ruth were married for twenty-four years, and she was a blessing. I believe her strength and emotional health truly saved our family. She showered us with love and urged us to feel compassion for Dad; over time we all loved her back. For most of that time I lived in Illinois and came home to see her.

Dad continued to do what he had always done by staying involved in the community and helping others. He was a president or a member of numerous boards and groups, including his church, Boy Scouts, Kiwanis and others. He received the Jefferson Award for Public Service, a high honor, for his work establishing and acting as scoutmaster for twenty-seven years of a Boy Scout troop for disabled children at Gaenslen School in Milwaukee. He shepherded one boy to Eagle rank. I now understand that he did so much for so many essentially for two reasons: he believed it was the right thing to do, and the doing of it gave him praise for his work and the affirmation from others of his quality that his parents had never given him.

Maintaining the family facade didn't work for the rest of us. My brother, sister, and I drifted apart, each of us immersed in our own grief. My sister Peg, age fourteen, stayed in her room with the door closed. My brother Don, sixteen, seemed to make himself scarce. I suddenly felt completely alone and adrift in a world stripped of the old assumptions. All I had been taught about life and living – the importance of family and good deeds, honor and hard work to receive God's grace -- shattered in the instant of knowing she was gone. Mom's death skewed how I saw the world and myself.

The family collapsed emotionally, leaving me feeling abandoned with anger and grief as my companions. I was just a kid and couldn't understand or accept the loss of my mother. What I had been taught about life had been suddenly stripped away. My childhood joy evaporated. I didn't know who to blame, so naturally I blamed Dad.

At the time of Mom's death, I was involved in our church as an acolyte and a teacher for Sunday School and Vacation Bible School. I believed a white-bearded white man sat on a throne in heaven and thundered biblical justice on naughty children. I had been taught to face any problem or fear by praying and God would watch over me and bestow comfort and blessings. But that simple faith couldn't answer why such a terrible thing could descend on such an upright family, and why I hurt so badly. Our pastor could only answer with, "God works in mysterious ways." "Bullshit" came to my juvenile mind.

I lost my faith in church and God. I have tried over the years to renew it, but I've never recovered it. Why not? It made no sense to me why some good people like my mother die young, why a supposedly benevolent God could allow pain, suffering, and evil to flourish. I'm older now and educated enough to know that philosophers have been debating these issues for thousands of years, yet I still feel some deep anger about the seeming unfairness and unpredictability of it all.

But at age ten I didn't know the right words to ask and answer such questions. When the pillars of my support – church and mother – kicked over, I became very afraid. I grew afraid of uncertainty because the old ways didn't seem to work anymore. All I had was myself, and that wasn't enough for a kid. My fear grew in time to include people, intimacy, anything unknown, any kind of change. My fear of the dark grew into night terrors that have never completely left me.

***

Most children believe everything is alive. I sure did. I used to lie on the front lawn and daydream looking into hazy skies on long, hot, humid afternoons. My mind lifted up to the scudding clouds in a pale blue sky, where I watched dragons and birds mold and shift shapes just for me. I loved it then and still like to study the clouds for friendly shapes.

I knew that our house was alive. Our two-story brick house dozed quietly in the sun, but after dark I could hear the walls creak and groan as thunder growled in the wind. On such nights, alone in my second-floor bedroom, I knew something scary rustled in the attics all around me.

Every night I was sent to bed earlier than Don, which of course made sense because he was older. Some evenings the family would watch something scary on TV, and I'd beg Dad to let me stay up later, but he always refused. Rules are rules and must be obeyed. I had some comfort knowing that my brother would come to bed sometime later. That changed when Don was in the hospital with polio, and for the first time I felt completely alone up there.

After being ordered to go to bed, I'd walk slowly up the

stairs, counting as I climbed . . . 14, 15, and 16. I'd stop at the landing where the stairs reached the second floor. There was a window above the landing next to a door which opened onto the second-story rear porch.

In daytime, everything upstairs appeared normal and comfortable-- a bathroom on the left painted in bright blue, brownish carpet running the full length of the hallway, and pictures hanging along the walls; many of them were Native American art Dad had bought during family trips to Arizona and Utah. At the end of the hallway was another staircase descending to the front entryway. Nice colors in yellow, light green, and beige.

There were three attics in our house, two of which were near the landing. The one on the left stored Dad's fishing and hunting gear, and I'd take my friends in there to sneak peeks at the guns and other man-stuff. The attic to the right was used for storing of Christmas lights and decorations, luggage, and my great-grandfather Adolf's old-style, glass-faced banker bookcases packed with old books and encyclopedias. This attic was big, with enough odd corners to be a great place for hide-and-seek.

The third attic, the one at the end of the hall across from my bedroom, was different. There was an odd feel about it, a prickle of fear that whispered, "Don't come in here." That attic was the largest of the three; L-shaped with three curtained windows overlooking the front of the house. It had one dim yellowish bulb too weak to shed light in the dark corners. A green curtain hung over the window on the hallway side. Sometimes I'd be out in front of the house or across the street and look up at those three windows, and by a trick of the eye I'd know that curtain moved.

I stood on that landing, night after night, sometimes for an hour or more, staring down that hallway straining to hear any sound of what might lay in wait behind that curtain and the other attic doors.

"Help me," I'd called downstairs, "Help me, please" (But never too loudly, because I also feared Dad's anger). I'd call again, whispering the words like a suffocating man, but no one ever came.

I stood there, my heart beating like a drum, my body embalmed in fear. I knew deep down that no one would help me, that I was totally alone. The only way I could get down that hallway and into my bedroom was to recite the Twenty-third Psalm, three, five, even ten times, which would put me in a kind of trance so I could walk past those attic doors. It took every ounce of courage I had, every time, to overcome my terror.

I'd finally enter the bedroom and walk to the nightstand and turn on the old red-tube radio to listen to fifties tunes or a Braves baseball game. I quickly slid under the covers and pulled the sheet tight over my head; no skin could show, that might invite something I didn't want to think about. I made sure that my feet never hung over the side.

My bed sat under three windows, two of which were always open wide to beckon any stray draft of air to bring relief from the summer heat and humidity. I'd lay only on my left side facing the windows and away from the door, my ears perked for any sound, scratch or breath. Sweat rolled down my back as the shade slapped lazily in the heavy air. I'd squeeze my eyes tight trying to make my mind go blank. I could never sleep because my mind was on full alert for any sound. But I'd fake being asleep when Don came to bed, and only then could I fall asleep.

For years I've tried to find adequate words to describe the fear I felt looking down that hallway – terror maybe, but none I can think of seem deep or broad enough. My fear abated in high school because I was older, but also out of necessity. That bedroom became my refuge. It was my runaway place inside the house.

That fear scarred me so deeply that it has never disappeared.

I feel the willies when I'm alone in dark places. Some of that fear may be normal human survival instinct from the days when humans were prey to fanged animals. Camping alone, though, keeps my heart pumping and ear cocked to hear the slightest sound. I always close our bedroom door when my wife Rene is gone; I don't sleep well with an open door. I have to turn a light on to make a bathroom run.

***

I've done inner child work on this fear in various healing groups and that has helped me a lot. The inner child, as a "metaphorical me," helped me to explore my deepest feelings. Early on I could close my eyes and imagine my kid hiding inside a cage and looking out with his hands grasping the iron bars.

My kid showed up one day when I was writing this section and trying to put words to the fear and the sense of being totally alone when confronting that hallway. I saw him hanging around that cage again. Take my hand, I said, and I'll walk with you down that hallway and tuck you in. Then you can tell me your scary fears, and I'll tell you mine. And then, together, we'll let them go and we won't have to feel afraid anymore.

Now he runs free, but I still shiver a bit in the dark.

***

My sister Peg and I have always been close, each of us succoring and supporting the other through good times and bad. Especially the bad. A catastrophe struck in 1976 that nearly destroyed us. Peg's first-born, Elaine, was diagnosed at age six with an inoperable brain tumor, and eventually died. Those six months, from diagnosis to funeral, were a special level of hell for me, and all of us, as we watched powerless as the cancer sucked the life out of this precious girl.

I was living in central Illinois at the time and drove to Milwaukee every weekend knowing there was nothing I could say or do but sit with Peg so she could vent rage at the horrible unfairness of it all. In answer to "Why?" I heard, "God works in mysterious ways," from Peg's pastor. "Bullshit," was our joint answer.

The little hope and faith in the future I still held after Mom's death died with my niece. The commandments I had grown up with—work hard, have faith in the future, trust in God and all will be well—were lies. I had all the proof I needed that betrayal was the way of the world, and nothing mattered. I was fucked.

I had always been a euphoric drinker, eager for the sense of well-being I'd find in the bottle, and I kept some of that to my last drink. But after that ghastly day, booze no longer pushed the darkness away. My drinking turned pathological, and I abandoned all hope that my life might get better. I drank for another nine years, becoming a nihilistic, fatalistic, hopeless drunk filled with anger. I started thinking about buying a gun.

***

My brother Don was an excellent student, who went to an excellent undergraduate college, majored in chemistry (much to Dad's delight) and went on to earn a Ph.D. in chemistry and land an important job with an international chemical company. By comparison, I was wandering in a wilderness of bad choices.

My response to his achievements was fueled by my lingering anger that he had stolen my spotlight after his hospital stay. I was intensely jealous of his success, and I tried to wound him, not to his face, of course; by spewing my contempt for those who had "sold out" to the corporate world to anyone who would listen. "Look at me," I'd say, "I haven't taken the bait and live a real life." That life of mine filled a bottle and nothing more.

I lived in illusion and couldn't admit that my life was my responsibility, that I had sold my soul to Johnnie Walker and his comrades. I sanctimoniously claimed my lousy life was caused by a conspiring world that awarded the lucky ones (everyone else) and failed the deserving (me).

Don and I spent many long years with little contact, but we're both working to change that, finally.

Full of fear and frustration because, God forbid, as a kid I couldn't fight Dad or his rules, I started beating up my friends. I'd throw a punch in a flash, then hear their cries and beg their forgiveness. I'd plead with them to hit me back as hard as they could, thinking I was offering justice. This cycle repeated itself for years – I got angry when friends wouldn't do what I needed them to do and explode, then whimper.

In my teens Boy Scouts was my life saver. I joined a troop headed by two scoutmasters who insisted all twenty-four of us work for Eagle rank, and they tried to take all of us on an outing every month. We went on long hikes, sometimes twenty-five miles in two days in other states. We also took a few lengthy canoe trips in the Boundary Waters and northern Wisconsin. Dad rarely came on those trips, so for a weekend or longer I felt emancipated from his rules.

By assuming the role of eager beaver, I created my own rules. I'd portage a canoe then go back and haul two Duluth packs. I was the troop's woodchopper. I helped maintain order by warning the older boys to stop bullying the younger. I became my father and got affirmed for the same reason; I needed it and lapped it up like a kitten with a bowl of cream. Then back home to my victimhood.

Trying to follow in Dad's footsteps I often became even more rigid then he was. In the summer of 1966, for example, I was a merit badge counselor at a Boy Scout camp outside Milwaukee.

I warned all the Scouts seeking camping merit badges that they had to do the required tent set-up and campfire cooking as well as answer correctly every question required, no exceptions.

One Scout from an Illinois troop worked hard and had completed the requirements for the camping merit badge but failed to answer one question correctly. I self-righteously denied him the badge, which infuriated his scout leaders who complained to the camp directors. It was a sick and lousy thing I did to that boy – I took revenge on that innocent youth for what I felt was always being done to me -- and thankfully the camp awarded him the merit badge.

I also found solace in music. As a kid I always flipped through Dad's large collection of jazz and classical LPs. Big Band music – Basie, Ellington, Armstrong – was Dad's favorite, and my ears perked up when classical was on the hi-fi. Beethoven and Mozart were my first music loves. I had to take piano lessons because Don and Peg took them, and from the same piano teacher, too. I hated the idea just for that reason and deliberately made mistakes, which I paid for sometimes with Mom's thimble-rapping my head. To be honest, I had a great ear for music but little skill at it. Even on days when I was alone and tinkled the keys, I heard music in my head that my fingers couldn't play.

My family story would be incomplete without some stories about Norma, Dad's mother, the scourge of the family.

My mother's parents, Wall and Cora, could also have posed for Norman Rockwell. They lived in a tidy home with built-in bookshelves framing a fireplace, Grandpa's rocking chair set to one side and pies on the table. They died within a year of each other when I was eight, so my memories of them are thin.

Any history of alcoholism in my family probably starts with my other grandfather, Gallus, Dad's father. Dad obviously had issues with alcohol – one drink only at a sitting was his rule. Genetics has a role to play. Family heredity studies reveal that as much as one half of a person's risk of becoming addicted to alcohol depends on genetic makeup. Dad wasn't a drunk, but I sure am, and it might be my inheritance from his father. (See Note 6 for more about genetics and addiction.)

Gallus was a rascally character. He liked to drink and gamble, but he loved fishing most of all. Our neighbor Don, a boyhood friend of Dad's, told us how often times he'd walk down the alley to pick up Dad for school and hear Grandpa snoring in the car in the garage.

I remember going out fishing with him when I was maybe four years old. He often spanked me for toddling on his worm patch. He rousted me up before dawn, and the two us climbed into the old wooden fishing boat and oared out on the lake. He'd drop the anchor, dump a net full of beer bottles over the side, and say these words: "We're not moving, so no complaining, and if you have to go, either one or two, over the side." Then he'd drop his line in the water.

The man could catch fish where nobody else could. On a wall in my college dorm room, I hung up a pipe rack he'd made on which he'd mounted the head of the biggest northern pike ever caught in that lake. Its long, sharp teeth guarded my roommates' bags of weed and hash.

I have a picture of him sitting at a table in the backyard at the lake. He has a cigarette in hand and a "Don't fuck with me" glare on his face. He had this expression in several other pictures of him that I have, and you can tell by the look in his eyes that this was not a pleasant guy. Even so, I really enjoyed reading to him when he lay paralyzed and dying from Lou Gehrig's disease.

Which brings me to his wife, my Grandmother Norma. What to tell? She dressed Dad in a suit and sent him out to play with the other boys. If he came home dirty, he got spanked, bathed, and dressed in another suit and sent back outside. She had specially made tin cups with wrist chains to cover his hands so he couldn't chew his fingernails. She was obsessive about cleanliness; she kept more than a dozen pails, each labelled for one particular job and no other. Each pail had its own set of boiled, iron rags. She could charm the pants off anyone, but she was cold as a lizard and as self-centered as Narcissus.

I wanted her to die for how she treated my mother. She treated my mother horribly, and I'll probably never forgive her for that. Mom, in pain from the cancer, stayed in Norma's second bedroom at the lake. Mom was always uncomfortable because the August nights that summer were hot and humid and there was no air conditioning in her room. There was only one fan, which Grandma didn't want to surrender. She also made sure to keep the TV volume loud, and when Mom asked her to turn it down, Norma told us (this I remember): "I can't even do what I want in my own house."

Over the years I've prayed and found some empathy for her, because it seemed obvious that something had been done to her as a child. Every therapist and psychiatrist I've seen has said that child abuse could explain her behavior. That could be the case, but it's impossible to know. I will admit I've struggled to have empathy for her even forty plus years after she died. She was such a powerful presence etching so many memories in our brains that when Don, Peg and I got together years ago, we regaled ourselves by telling stories of Norma's nastiness. We're finally moving past that.

That is my family, a short profile of its personalities, struggles, and oddities. I certainly played a role in its dysfunction, and I no longer can blame anyone but myself for my part in causing much of it. We all were products of our time and cultural heritage, cursed by family tragedy, pain, and confusion. All of us, Dad included, ached for some sense of normality, chaining ourselves to the usual routines to face a world that had totally changed. Don, Peg, and I acted in ways to defend us from the pain and make sense of it all. I chose alcohol.

PART II:
MY ROADMAP TO HEALING

*The secret of health for both mind and body is not to mourn for
the past, not to worry about the future, nor to anticipate troubles,
but to live in the present moment wisely and earnestly.*
--Buddha

Part I told of my slide into the alcohol pit and being rescued by
AA and treatment. Part II tells of the specific things I had to do,
and continue doing, to build and enrich my sobriety. I talk of how
nature helped me find my true self; how therapy and my psycholo-
gist wife helped me uncover deep grief that clouded my heart. And
I describe some of my character defects that I need to work on.

***

I started drinking young and turned into a near-suicidal drunk
when a miracle saved me, epiphanies encouraged me, and good
luck plus hard work made me the man I am today. I found friends
in AA that I could trust who told me things about myself that I
usually didn't want to hear. My friends helped me to find the courage I needed to dig out my secrets, get honest, and change my
thinking.

It took me a while to appreciate how at ease I felt being around
other AA members which helped me realize how similar I was to
the people I met there. I had a good sponsor who patiently listened
to my complaints but gave me stern feedback. AA friends told me
their truths. I sought therapy when I needed help. I became willing, finally, to work the 12 Steps as best I could.

I learned to honor myself and others, accept my non-sainthood and begin to live a life worth living. I had to honor the fear, pain, and love in my core and flush out the bullshit. I came to know the happiness of honesty and the freedom of dancing to my own music. To get there I had to forgive myself and get honest about the pain I caused. For that I needed the 12 Steps as a guide. Following the Steps began my healing.

CHAPTER 9

THE TWELVE STEPS

Removing old conditionings from the mindand training the mind to be more (calmness) with every experience is the first step enabling one to experience true happiness.
--S.N. Goenka, Indian meditation teacher

What follows is my history with the 12 Steps, both in the past and as they continue to unfold in my life. I struggled with some of them, no question. There's no specific order to my work on these; and my understanding of each Step came when I was open to its message, quickly with some and slowly with others. As I've grown in age and sobriety, my understanding of them has changed and deepened, just as red cherry wood over time turns a lustrous deep red-orange brown.

AA co-founder Bill Wilson first wrote the Steps in 1935 with the idea of making them mandatory for recovery. AA's first members, remembering their past rebellions against being told what to do, convinced him to adopt "a suggested program of recovery." A wise choice, because otherwise I would have flushed the Big Book down the toilet.

An interesting thing about these Steps: Alcohol is mentioned only in the First and Twelfth Steps. The other ten Steps focus on particular things to do to help change how we think about ourselves and our behavior toward others. I needed to make those changes if I wanted to stay sober.

Step One: We admitted we were powerless over alcohol, and that our lives had become unmanageable. I entered AA an adult man stuck in emotional toddlerhood knowing I had to quit drinking but not believing I was an alcoholic. I was a three-year-old in a thirty-seven-year-old body, waiting for someone to play my sister's role and do what I wanted. "King Baby" is a common term used to describe guys like me.

Many of the stories I heard others tell were wildly outside my experience – theft, gun battles, jail time and more. That convinced me I was way better than them. I, on the other hand, had a home, and a job with good salary so I could afford a car, fancy clothes, and huge restaurant and bar bills. By comparison with people I came to know at AA, I was near the top of the hill when I quit drinking, a long way above the gutter into which others had slid.

At heart I was just a scared kid who had never grown up and needed some kind of control over people and things to feel safe. I always thought I could control the next thing that came along, so the idea of surrendering and admitting my powerlessness over people, places, and things was incomprehensible to me – and terrifying. If I couldn't control what was going on around me, then anything could happen. I couldn't handle that idea, so what did I do? I erased from my daily life people and things that wouldn't do my bidding. I lived in a very small world.

My sponsor Ron challenged my denial of this First Step. Was my life a mess? Could I really control my drinking? How was my life going?

Of course, I responded with, "I could stop whenever I wanted to. I just didn't want to."

He laughed. "Then why are you here? It's obvious you couldn't control your drinking, so think of alcohol as a power greater than you," he said.

Over time I came to understand that my life was indeed a miserable mess because of drinking which induced me to do some stupid and terrible things. It took months of daily, sometimes twice-daily meetings listening to others tell their stories to grasp how crazy my life really was, the costs I had paid, and the damage I had inflicted on others. It took even more time for me to see that I had no power over other people or things. I can only control my own thinking and behavior.

Step Two: Came to believe that a power greater than ourselves could restore us to sanity.

I didn't understand what a "power greater than myself" should look like or actually be. I had been mentally pushing back against God and powerful people – including Dad and Don and various bosses -- almost my whole life. I believed religion was a farce, and the idea of surrendering to such a power was unthinkable. I insisted that I was not insane, because everyone else was.

It wasn't until I entered treatment that I began to see how I had martyred myself with self-pity from the stories I had created about myself, that I wasn't smart, I was a fraud and born to be a failure. This was the awakening of sanity in my adult life, the first ray of honesty when I began to see the world not as I wanted it to be but how it really is. It helped me turn -- slowly, for sure -- toward making honesty a habit and responsibility a necessity.

The folks sitting around those tables in AA who spoke truly about their own struggles led me to develop ("cultivate," as Old Timer Bill always said) a sense of gratitude for everything in my life, both the good and not-so good. The AA program and the people helped me find a sense of well-being that I had been seeking for a long time.

Step Three: Turned our will and our lives over to the care of God as we understand him.

I have long struggled with this one. I had told myself for decades that religion and God were nothing but a hypocritical scam on the weak minded. It wasn't for several years, after a stint in treatment and thousands of meetings, that my mind shifted like a compass point to a new direction.

I came to believe that nurturing a sense of serendipity, "The art of finding good things unlooked for," creates the magic of life. All I needed to do was open my heart and invite it in. Some may call that God's Grace descending, but I believe differently and no longer argue about it.

I now believe that I stand in a living river that always flows, wide or narrow depending on my mood, and is filled with all kinds of good things ready for my choosing. I spent my drinking life believing I stood in a desert with blinders to block the light and only look down. My sobriety deepened when I chose to throw those blinders away and wade in.

That set the table for the second most dramatic event of my life. (November 2, 1985, the day of the Miracle, was the first, and remains the greatest.)

After I quit my job as a liquor salesman in June 1989, I felt a deep need to see the West again. I was four years sober and yearned to see again the red rocks, cactus, and canyons I treasured in memory from long-ago family vacations. I have a photo of me at about six years old standing on the rim of the Grand Canyon wearing a cowboy hat, huge smile and toy pearl-handled six-shooters. I decided to go for it and planned a six-week trip to Arizona, Utah, and Colorado in summer 1989. It was a trip that reshaped my life.

My life-changing moment occurred when I was camped in Monument Valley on the Navajo Nation. I remembered that place from John Huston westerns, especially Stagecoach, and old vacation pictures and Arizona Highways magazines my father collected. There was something vital I couldn't yet define about those buttes, spires, and colors, but I felt drawn, even coaxed, by something outside myself to stay by them.

I staked my tent there for three days and watched and listened, trying to take it all in. I stood in awe of the rose-colored sky over the Mittens and Merrick Butte. I explored some in the valley, but for three days I sat on a ledge as an observer, distinct and distant, looking at that land's texture, color and vastness as if I was sitting in an art gallery.

That changed on the third day. I was sitting in my chair looking at the Valley when another of the many epiphanies (the promised magic) I've had in sobriety shattered my isolation. One second changed me forever.

I don't remember anything in particular that sparked this epiphany, but in one instant I felt alone and separate from everything before me, and in the next I suddenly knew in my gut that I was a part of this place, that I was embraced by everything in this world. My fear of always being alone was swept away like dust in a freshening wind. The voluptuousness of the place embraced me, and tears flooded my eyes. My heart danced to a very different tune, like a long-lost childhood song I now heard once more. It was a mind blow that started healing my spirit.

I luxuriated in that place for a couple more days and drove to Longmont, Colorado, to visit a friend. A few days later I started for home, and the minute I entered I-80 heading east I started sobbing. My tears just flowed for no reason I could think of. I didn't feel sorry or sad or angry or frustrated. I was just awash in tears whose source I didn't understand; I knew I had changed in some fundamental ways but didn't fully understand how much. I cried continuously for the two days it took to drive back to Milwaukee.

One night I stayed in Des Moines and called my next-door neighbor, Jim. I tried to explain that I didn't feel sad or any other emotion, that all I did all day was cry. The next morning, I bought a latte and re-entered I-80 and I cried all the way back home in Milwaukee. Jim helped me to understand that I was undergoing an emotional purge of my sick soul and re-connecting my heart with long-lost love of the outdoors. No wonder those tears felt like a cleansing.

The next day I pulled into my driveway in Milwaukee and Jim walked over and gave me a huge bear hug. Jim and his wife Kay were deeply pious, earthy people who I had adopted as my spiritual advisers. Jim handed me an article from Christian Century magazine entitled "Fierce Landscapes and the Indifference of God" by Belden C. Lane. Read this, he said, and maybe it'll help you understand what you just went through. I did, and it did.

Lane, a theologian, argues that fierce landscapes, indifferent to petty wants and needs, break our egos and offer a path to spirituality and a sense of the divine. Jim said my tears showed I had probably experienced that very thing. As Lane put it, "In the frightening experience of having our fragile egos ignored, we are thrust beyond fear to grace unexpected."

I read it and came away confirmed that my experience in Monument Valley with the rocks, trees, wind, and sky was the key to my healing.

Step Four: Made a searching and fearless moral inventory of ourselves.

I first worked on this step when I was in treatment. I had started rewriting my autobiography (as explained above), and for the first time, I tried to be honest about my drinking and past behavior. I came to understand that I did such things because I was drinking, and now that I was sober, I could stop doing that kind of stupid shit.

It took some time for that to sink in. I had been running from the truth for so long that lashing myself seemed a normal and just punishment. Regretting what I had done was one thing, but I wallowed in that guilt, and that was something else again. I had to admit that I gloried in my misbehavior – "See what I did? Try and beat that!"

Starting this Step, I knew I had to write down and take responsibility for the emotional abuse I had inflicted on the woman I married in 1980, five years before I quit drinking.

I first knew Angie (not her real name) when I was head bartender at a pizza joint in Milwaukee. It was in 1971, and she was dating Pat, who was a regular with his friend Larry. She was a beautiful party gal with a loud voice, coarse language, and suggestive eye. I fell in lust. Nothing happened...yet. A few years later, I moved to central Illinois and managed a deli owned by two brothers, my friends. In 1979 Angie called me from Milwaukee and offered to come by train for a visit. I met her at the Champaign, Illinois, train station, and within an hour we were drinking and in bed. A wild weekend followed of drinking and sex, then she went back to Milwaukee. I decided to follow her.

I stayed with Dad and Ruth in my old bedroom. Angie and her daughter lived with her sister. Angie and I would go out for an evening of drinking and horseplay and get a room at a Ramada Inn. One night, after drunken sex, I proposed to her. She said yes.

The next morning at home, I woke up with a terrible headache and dread: "Oh man, what did I do?" I knew the marriage would never work, but I didn't have the balls to tell Angie that the booze was talking, that we needed to hold off and think about it. It was easier to go ahead with wedding plans and cover my misgivings, as always, with bravado.

"Bob, are you sure you want to do this?" someone asked me.

"I don't know if it will work, but I'm willing to try anything once," I said trying to sound super-cool. "If not, I'll just get divorced."

Everyone around me knew I was making a huge mistake, but I ignored them. Why? If I admitted I was making a mistake, the blustery tough facade I maintained for everyone else would crumble. And I simply couldn't risk that. I ignored my gut feelings and pushed ahead with the wedding plans.

The big day arrived, and at 11 a.m. I stood at the altar badly hung over from an all-night drunken stag party. We said our vows, everyone had some nice food, and we took off for an evening of drinking and passed out at our new apartment.

I made sure that things went downhill from there. I acted passive aggressively about nearly everything. I argued about simple things like folding towels, washing dishes, household chores. Angie wanted things done a certain way, but I made a point of quarreling over everything.

Why did I act like that? I know now I resented her for agreeing to marry me, for demanding I be the good husband I didn't really want to be. I wanted to do what I wanted when I wanted, and she could take care of herself and leave me alone. I felt disgusted with my lack of courage and marrying her, so I lashed out at her by trashing the commitment I made at the altar. One night, Angie asked me if I would be willing to adopt her daughter, and I said: "I'd prefer to wait to make sure this works." That badly hurt her, but I didn't care.

I made myself the victim by bitching to everyone about how she was driving me crazy with towel folding and dish rinsing. I used that to excuse my first extra-marital affair that I made happen about thirty days after the altar. I used the same excuse to walk out on her three months later. I stayed with a friend for a couple of weeks; Angie and I reconciled, and I moved back in. I left for good in another two months, saw an attorney, told him I wanted a divorce and to give her everything. A judge granted it in February 1982. I was free again.

I prided myself on living on the edge, willing to take risks no one else would, that I was something special for laying waste to others' well-being. I had a perverse feeling that I had finally achieved something in life – notoriety, perhaps – in contrast to my straightlaced father and brother.

Now sober, writing these things down has opened my mind to just how awful I had been to them and others. But I took a perverse turn by cloaking myself in a new notoriety and flagellating myself for all to see. "See what I've done" now became, "See how much more a badass I am than you." I felt proud of myself.

There were many things I did to other people on my list – verbal back-stabbings, lies and manipulations – but none matched what I had inflicted on her. My list grew longer the deeper I dug. I had to write several Fourth Steps to get clear and honest about all I had done. Then I had to somehow agree to forgive myself. That wasn't easy.

Step Five: Admitted to God, to ourselves and another human being the exact nature of our wrongs.

I shared my Fourth Step story with Father G. while in treatment. I confessed my sins for more than an hour, verbally flagellating myself for my transgressions, when he yawned. How dare he! Doesn't he understand the importance of what I am telling him? That he was facing the worst person of all?

It was only later when I understood that my story was rather ho-hum compared to the mayhem of others' lives, and I had to deal with my conceit and narcissism. I still lacked a spiritual sense that could help me reach outside myself to have empathy for myself and others and grow into the fullness of being. Telling someone else what I had done helped move me out of the shadows. For some of that I would need therapy, and a lot of it. I had to learn how to cultivate humility, a rather alien concept at the time, and it slowly grew in me with work and self-reflection, beginning with Step Six.

Step Six: Were entirely ready to have God remove all these defects of character.

I didn't work this step for a long time because I was afraid to. I didn't want to let go of my defects. I had lived with them for so long that they had become my only identity. The ability to look someone straight in the eye and lie my pants off; emotional vampirism, leeching off the good will of others; verbal bullying; envy and resentment inflamed with passive-aggressiveness. I had no idea who I was or could be without those defects of character, so I held on tight.

My AA friends Tom and Nona helped by opening me up to new ideas and possibilities, and challenging me to be honest about my behavior, past and present, and change my attitude towards people and life. They didn't tolerate my bullshit. Jim and Kay, my neighbors, didn't either.

I spent a lot of time talking with Jim and Kay sitting around their kitchen table. Amid the chitchat about news and books, they challenged my self-perceptions and helped me to understand and share their belief that an all-encompassing faith in the possibility of good in the world could change my life. They taught me to see the glass as half full, not half empty.

Jim and Kay, with Tom and Nona, helped to make me a spiritual man open to the epiphanies and awakenings that were to come. They affirmed me as a basically good person despite screwed-up thinking, especially what I thought about myself. They hugged me when I needed it most. I responded to them as a puppy does to a good scratching.

Step Seven: Humbly asked Him to remove our shortcomings

I didn't like the wording of this step because it smacked too much of church and religion. I had come to want change, and I wanted to become a better man, but I was still holding on to my old ways.

This Step presented me with a very important question: If I let go of my shortcomings, who will I be?

To answer that I had to find some trust and faith that the sobriety I was working for would give me all that it promised. I needed help with that and asked for help from my friends. They told me about their hopes and dreams, which helped me open a door to a deeper understanding of who I could be. They helped me to see what I had to do – get more honest, let all my secrets out and then let them go.

Step Eight: *Made a list of all persons we had harmed and became willing to make amends to them all.*

When we got to this step my sponsor said he wanted my name at the top of the list. I didn't get it. You hurt yourself more than anyone else, he told me. I did it but didn't yet believe I deserved that because for some screwy reason I cherished wielding the whip to sanctify my suffering.

I put my first wife Angie and my father on that list, along with my sister, brother and friends. Of course, still damning myself, I added every shrug or side-swipe word I had ever used against anyone that I could remember. The list was long.

I learned a little about honesty and being responsible in the Fourth Step, but writing this list was different matter entirely. This Step was not an arms-length writing exercise but an actual listing of those I had to tell my faults to and ask forgiveness. It was a scary thing for me to bare my faults to others, but I did it. It took some bravery I didn't know I had, and I felt good in honestly doing it.

Step Nine: *Made direct amends to such people wherever possible, except when to do so would injure them or others.*

I turned to this next Step and immediately knew I had to make personal amends to Angie. Everyone around me, however, said I had no right to crash back into her life. Remember the second phrase, they said. They suggested I write a letter asking her forgiveness and then burn it. So that's what I did. It didn't feel quite complete then and still doesn't today. There is nothing else I can do.

I met with everyone on my list. In almost every case, I explained my behavior as a result of drinking, and said I wanted to apologize for any hurt I may have caused. I was met with surprise and almost instant forgiveness. And no wonder. I didn't let anyone get close enough to really know me. I was usually showed my calm and cool side and saved the dark one for the ballfield.

The typical response was, "Thanks for telling me. I've always wondered just what went wrong with you," or, "Oh, that was nothing, I forgot that long ago." The father of a childhood friend that I often bullied, said, "Of all the boys, you had the brains, intelligence and personality, and I've always wondered what the hell happened to you."

The friends I beat up when we were kids knew who I was back then and weren't nearly so forgiving. I accepted that.

Step Ten: Continued to take personal inventory and when we were wrong, promptly admitted it

I practice this step daily, and over time it's become an instinctual practice. I know in my gut when I'm not acting right; it's like an ethical ESP squad calling me to stop what I have just started and do something about it.

Of course, I'm sometimes deaf to that call, but healthy people in my life, especially my wife Rene, will ring it for me. Rene will not tolerate my thoughtlessness and acting out. She does it with firmness and love, and I usually don't like it at first. But I end up being thankful for her critique which helps me become more aware of things -- at least for a while.

The first time I practiced this Step was in Fall 1986 after I left treatment. I was back to work at my liquor sales job. One day I called Bea, the credit manager, to ask that a customer with an iffy payment history be allowed to purchase a large order. Bea had a small statue on her desk of a hand with an erect middle finger, and the words: "Our credit policy."

She said no, and I blew up and said some unpleasant things and slammed down the pay phone. I walked a few steps toward my car and stopped. I knew I had been an ass and had to call back and apologize. "Oh Bob, no problem at all. I hear it all the time," she laughed.

I felt grateful for her generosity but knew I had done the right thing. It was a new experience for me, and it felt great.

Step Eleven: Sought through prayer and meditation to improve our conscious contact with God as we understood him, praying only for knowledge of His will for us and the power to carry that out

I don't follow this step as written. I don't pray to God or meditate by sitting in a rigid pose with eyes closed and focused breathing. That works wonders for many of my friends, and I'm happy for them. I find a meditative mind in a forest, where sitting by a tree and just watching and listening really lights me up.

I learned to get on my knees and pray while in treatment, and I did it nightly for years after. Now I don't pray to the God of any religion; I seek communion with the Spirit I believe lives in everything by being outdoors. I pray to Spirit for forgiveness of my shortcomings and courage to open myself, and I find uplift in nature, Spirit incarnated.

Praying for me is an act of centering, of focusing, of saying out loud the wishes I have for myself. I don't ask for knowledge of Spirit's will, because I know my duty to my life, my wife and people I hold dear -- stay sober in body and grow in spirit. That's as clear to me as a bright star in the night sky.

Step Twelve: Having had a spiritual awakening as the result of these steps, we tried to carry this message to alcoholics and to practice these principles in all our affairs.

I always emphasize "spiritual experience as a result" when reading the Steps in a meeting. By the time I got to this one, I knew that being worthy of a life worth living requires that I be as honest as I can be and responsible for everything I do.

Along the way I learned that accepting my powerlessness over alcohol, people, places and things freed me from the self-imposed burden of trying to control everything. And accepting that I am not God (and no one else is, either) helped to erase my shame for being less-than. The work involved to stay sober freed me to walk open-eyed in the world.

I still attend AA meetings for my own mental health and to share my experience, strength, and hope with others about how I found sobriety. By giving of myself to someone else, I reap a harvest of well-being for myself. And I get blessings from folks who share their stories that encourage me to work harder to be a better man. I know this works, because over time I've sponsored many men who found new and exciting lives through working these Steps.

CHAPTER 10
HONESTY MATTERS

Growing up happens when you start having things you look back on and wish you could change.
--Cassandra Clare, American author

We defend ourselves by burying our traumatic events.
--Sigmund Freud

I like to imagine recovery work as a set of keys which I have used to unlock secrets and emotions hidden behind heavy, guarded doors. My first key unlocked a desire to stop practicing the addiction, and the second unlocked a willingness for change.

I needed a special key to unlock a particularly heavy door of my own -- this door I didn't want to open and, in fact, couldn't push it open without help from therapists. The stories I had been telling myself since childhood lay there behind the door, and I feared bringing them out. Other secrets lay hidden in shadows where I needed them to stay.

Twelve Step meetings are not therapy sessions. The Steps are guideposts on how to achieve clear thinking and good behavior, and we share with each other how we're doing, and offer our hope and experiences to those who are struggling. Many come to meetings knowing they're a safe place to share whatever terrible thing they're going through.

Exhuming the hidden stuff isn't easy, and getting honest about those memories can be even harder. In my case, the fellowship of meetings and the friends I met there comforted me enough to keep me from going back out. They promised that if I got some honesty and revealed my secrets, a door would open and my true self could join the light. They were right.

My own personal memories are of emotional trauma, not physical harm. Drinking is not kind to memory, and I didn't understand for a long time just how slippery some of my memories could be. In most cases decades of alcohol-fueled delusion warped my memories into a personal myth that distorted what really was.

I had to work hard on being honest about myself and my past and needed multiple therapies kick the door open and sweep out the shadows. I discovered while writing this book that, to my surprise, I still have a few more doors to open. (See chapter 12 for more on therapy.)

Working the Steps helped clear much of that out, but some powerful stuff remained, especially about my father and brother. The most important person I needed to be honest with was my father.

In 1993 I was eight years sober and knew I had to make amends with my father and share with him my truth about the pain and fear I felt growing up. I was living in Flagstaff, and he and his third wife, Mary, lived in Green Valley just south of Tucson. I feared confronting Dad but knew in my bones that I had to "stick my head in the dragon's mouth," as I put it. I met Cathy in Flagstaff, and she showed me how to do it.

That same year Cathy went into treatment in Tucson for relationship and eating disorders, and she invited me to attend the family weekend. Part of the treatment process was a two-day, mutual truth-telling in front of a group. The first day I told Cathy what I needed to say to her and she had to stay silent. The second day, I stayed silent while she talked. She and her mother did the same, and the other patients in turn interacted with their significant others.

I came away from that experience knowing I had to do the same thing with Dad. I had amends to make with him, but I also knew I had to confront him about the things he did and said to me when I was a kid. I was really scared to do it, because he was the center of my anger and love, the focus of my resentments and self-definition. I placed him on the highest pedestal of my imagining.

I told my men's group that I was going to do this, and they warned it was too dangerous for me to do such a thing alone. They volunteered to act as mediators, but I said no. "You don't understand, I have to do this." I was very anxious about doing this, but I later knew it was the bravest thing I had ever done or most likely will ever do. Our talking honestly with each other cleared the air between us and blessed us both. I somehow found the courage to state my truth and the miracle happened -- I gained what I had thrown away and was the man Dad thought he had lost. I became his loving son again and he my loving father.

I called him a day or two later and said I wanted to talk with him, just the two of us without Mary present.

"What do you want to talk about?" he asked.

"I'll explain when I get there," I said.

A long pause told me he was nervous. But he said OK. We set a date, and I prepared myself. I wrote him a long letter, laying down my amends and letting out the resentments and anger I had harbored for decades. I committed myself to getting it all out with him, to save myself. I burned the letter.

A few days later I drove to Green Valley and arrived at their house on time. No one was there, which surprised me. Dad was always prompt, calling it a sign of respect for the person he was meeting. He insisted us kids be prompt as well. Mary had left a note that Dad had gotten sick that morning, and she had taken him to the doctor. I stood at the front door as they drove up, with Dad slouched against the side door and looking unwell and ill at ease. We went inside, and Dad sat in his chair and I took the couch. He said he wasn't feeling well, and did I really want to do this today? I had a decision to make, an important one, and I somehow found the courage to say, Yes. Mary graciously left the house, and there we were, alone with each other.

I told Dad that I wanted to talk and asked him to just listen and not interrupt until I was done. Then I would listen to whatever he needed to say to me. I got a few words out … and he interrupted. "Dad, just listen to me, please, then I will listen to you," I said. And he agreed, I think reluctantly.

I talked maybe for two hours, the whole time in tears. I shared my anger over Mom's death, how he never seemed to recognize my individuality, and all the hurt I suffered from his mother. I told him how I had abused him behind his back, talked badly about him to my friends, how passive-aggressive I acted toward him, the blatant disregard I showed him when around others, his refusal to acknowledge and accept my alcoholism, and the list went on. I said how sorry I was for being so stupidly angry as a teenager all the time and asked for his forgiveness. I told him that despite everything, I had always loved him and now at long last wanted a loving, close relationship with him.

Finally, I was done, my face and shirt wet with tears. And then an amazing thing happened. Dad affirmed me, for the first time since I could remember. (He had probably done so many times before, but I closed my ears.) He stood up and sat beside me on the couch. He looked in my tear-swollen eyes and said, "It took a lot of guts to do what you just did."

Then he talked and I listened. He talked about how difficult his childhood had been, how he had sacrificed the university teaching job he loved to honor his father's dying request that he take over the book-binding business, and about wanting to shoot himself when it went belly-up in 1968. He talked about how much he loved Mom and that all he ever wanted was to protect us from the pain and fear of mother's cancer.

We hugged each other, both of us crying, for a long time. As I write this, I can feel tears welling up over how precious that time with him was. Those few hours with him stripped me clean of all the resentments against him I had carried for decades.

Our shared honesty, both of us lowering our masks, allowed him to change, too. I learned then that honestly sharing my secrets with another person frees them to unlock their own. I wanted the meeting and Dad met me half-way. We both grew with each other.

Dad invited me to stay overnight, but I chose to camp near the top of Mt. Lemon outside Tucson. I stood on a large rock facing the dying sun. I stretched my arms to the sky, yelled and cheered with my heart full of love for Dad and feeling free of all the crap I had carried for decades. I had lied and emotionally castrated myself with lies about Dad for too many years, and I didn't have to do that anymore. I was finally free.

Those few hours with Dad fundamentally changed our father-son relationship. I could caretake him when he was getting immobilized with Parkinson's and with love bathe, feed and watch over him. We talked more deeply with each other. I could hold him in my arms and tell him how much I loved him – and he told me the same. This, the man I had hated most of my life.

Many sober friends of mine didn't have this luxury, because when they were ready to do it a parent may have closed himself off, suffered from dementia, or died. Some put it off until it was too late. A few did the next best thing – they a wrote letter to a parent venting their anger at what had been done to them. Then they burned the letter in a rite of cleansing and release. Some others were hesitant to dredge up the awful memories they'd spent years burying, and didn't think the emotional cost was worth the effort. Over time I've found that most folks in recovery understand the importance of establishing the truth of their past and challenge, by letter or face-to-face, whatever or whoever needs to be confronted.

***

While writing that story I knew I also had to start anew with my brother. I always admired Don and felt a love that I tried to deny. We each have our own issues with each other, but I'm working to let my love shine through the old bullshit. The key for me is to let Don just be Don, flaws and all, just as I now allow myself to be me.

My first years in this world were molded by the undivided attention of my sister. I understood that Don, being the oldest kid, was entitled to certain privileges, including being in charge of Dad's Holy Grail, the front lawn. My self-inflicted problem with my brother was really a simple one: I placed him on a pedestal and never let him off.

I was jealous of his career and successes since I was a kid – don't younger brothers always put their older brothers on pedestals? The turning point for me was when Don came home from the hospital and my parents focused on him. They were worried about his recovery from polio, so no sports or traveling for him. I still wanted all the attention I was used to and blamed him for hogging my spotlight.

What I refused to acknowledge at the time, of course, was the very uninteresting life I had created for myself out of fear of taking a risk. I opted for careers in the liquor and restaurant industries instead of going to graduate school or trying new things. I stuck myself in mediocre careers which were of little interest to my relatives. Out of courtesy they would ask a perfunctory question, "What are you doing these days?" I'd start describing and they'd say, "Uh hunh," then turn to the crowd around Don, who regaled everyone with stories of foreign countries and large construction projects.

Over the years I liked being around Don but kept my distance. A couple of times I visited Don and his wife Kitty in Connecticut and cracked jokes, talked politics and sports, and drank fine wine. After I sobered up, I went East again and confronted Don about him not staying in touch with me. What I really wanted was his attention and affirmation which, to be honest, I didn't yet deserve. I was still in early recovery having done minimal inner work, so I couldn't yet account for my role in all of it.

We both made a start when I lived in Flagstaff. Don asked to come visit and go camping, and I said yes. We drove to Monument Valley on the Navajo reservation and then to Canyonlands National Park in southeastern Utah. Neither of us can remember how many days we camped or other places we visited, but we both remember sharing the wonder of the huge monoliths of weathered red sandstone carved by wind and water and washed with desert varnish. It is an amazing landscape that looks fierce but welcomes the open-hearted.

We sat on a ledge at Monument Valley – the same place where I sat on in 1989 -- looking at that fantastically beautiful and rugged place and started talking with each other. Don and I traditionally talk sports, politics, the latest news and tales of family craziness. But this time was different. I asked about Mom, and as it turns out neither of us have much memory of her. We talked of other things for sure, but they were probably about everyday kind of stuff that we don't remember. I fondly remember it as a great time together.

We hiked every day in the slick rock, stood in awe of how the wind and rain carved such beauty in the red rocks and gloried in the azure blue sky that followed us everywhere. A few days later Don flew back to his world and I stayed in mine.

Over the past twenty-odd years our connection has faded and come back. I went to graduate school and began a new career in journalism, and Rene suddenly appeared out of nowhere; another unexpected event that upended my life. Don and I reach out to each other by phone every once in a while, but I want more now that I fully understand my role in keeping our relationship distant.

CHAPTER 11

SOME OF WHAT I LEARNED

*Tell me, what is it you plan to do with your one wild
and precious life?*
--Mary Oliver, "The Summer Day"

It is never too late to be what you might have been.
--T.S. Eliot

The Steps and the process of making amends made clear that I had
much more work to do. After all, sobriety is an inside job, and I
had to dig in deeper.

Over time I learned the answers to some questions that had
haunted me in early sobriety. How am I going to live without alcohol? I've got to quit, but where does that leave me? Who am I
without what I've always believed about myself?

Finding answers to those existential questions wasn't easy.
I had to change how I saw myself and the world. The deeper I
searched inside myself, the more I experienced epiphanies. They
would come when least expected. Sometimes I'd go to bed thinking one way and wake up knowing a different path had appeared.

Here's what I needed to do, which I talk more about in following chapters:

• I sought therapy when I was emotionally stuck.

• I had to deal with unresolved grief.

• I cultivated gratitude.

• I found emotional comfort in the natural world.

• I learned to expect the unexpected.

• Delving into my past showed that my negative energy
attracted more of the same. That pattern reversed when I worked
to stay sober. *(See Note 11 for the science research.)*

CHAPTER 12
THERAPY

Only in the darkness can you see the stars.
--Martin Luther King, Jr.

Meetings offer advice and support, but so many of my emotional problems were outside the scope of AA and I needed outside help to deal with them.

I offer this example. I was nine years sober and working for a remodeling contractor in Flagstaff. My crew was in the middle of a winter remodeling of a lodge in the South Rim village of the Grand Canyon. One night I had the most riveting, powerful dream of my life. I woke from it and sat upright in bed covered with sweat. It felt like an electrical shock had zapped my body. I couldn't get that dream out of my mind for several weeks, and I finally asked a friend to recommend a therapist. Phyllis was her name.

At our first session, I told Phyllis my life story which, of course, I spun out like old familiar yarn. Going that way won't work very well, she said, so we'll try something different -- Guided Imagery. She had me sit erect on the couch with body relaxed and eyes closed. I was to describe whatever image came up when she asked me about a word or name. When she said "father," I replied, "giant with a smile." After more image and response, Phyllis said "mother," and Mom appeared. I guess I fell into a trance, because she appeared out of nothing and sat in front of me, looked me in the eye with her hands folded and smiled. And waited.

I mentioned earlier that I had kept few memories of my mother. I buried my anger about her dying and leaving me because I had heard over and over how like a saint she was, and how could

I be angry with a saint?

Now, in my mind, she was with me, and for the first time since the day of her death, I could tell her how angry I was that she left me without saying goodbye. She said she was sorry; her life had become so miserable that she had to leave, and the cancer was her only way out. I sat on that couch and sobbed; she said she loved me and faded from view.

Phyllis called to me and I emerged on the couch, my shirt soaked in tears. That session was a miracle of transformation that cleansed me of that anger I had buried when I was ten. I felt free again just as I had after my time with Dad.

There are other therapies that also helped me, in particular what's called the Tapping solution. It involves working with a therapist and lightly tapping with fingers on the Chinese meridian points on the face while speaking of an emotional issue. When my wife Rene first told me about it, as she's a practitioner, I thought it sounded like a lot of hoo-hah.

Nevertheless, I tried it once with Rene to address deep biases I have about wealth and (in my view) its vulgar display. Before we started, my emotional energy level was about 9; after several rounds of tapping, to my surprise, it had dropped to near zero. The lesson I learned from this? I can become a victim of my own thoughts, so better to think positively and let the rest of it go. I remind myself that we're not rich, but we live in great abundance.

CHAPTER 13
GRIEF UNFOUND

Grief is of two parts. The first is loss. The second is the remaking of life.
--Anne Roiphe, American journalist and novelist

There is no grief like the grief that does not speak.
--Henry Wadsworth Longfellow, American poet

My journey with grief started after the Miracle knocked me dry and I chose to get sober. I was a twisted, angry man before that happened and completely out of touch with the emotional baggage I had lugged around for decades.

My first step was to listen to the advice of a psychiatrist I saw when I was in treatment. She said dabbing paint on a canvas might help me drill below my brain and into my gut where the emotions lie. I needed to get in touch with all my emotions, she said, to flush out the fear and anger that created my emotional constipation. I took her advice.

I don't remember all the details, but I purchased some acrylic paints, brushes, and paper. The instructor showed me the basics – whitewash the page, use a fan brush to squiggle distant pine tree branches, and mix colors to shade mountain crags. I instantly loved doing it and stuck around for more sessions.

When those ended, I was eager to do more of it, so I bought an easel and set it up in my bedroom. One day I just started swathing paint on the canvas, my mind rather blank to any idea and just following a whim. A shape took form. Intrigued, I brushed around that shape, and what emerged was an amorphous figure in brown slumped over and resting on a green slab. The more I stared at the image, the more clearly I saw a man bent over, arms on knees, with his hands cradling the back of his head. I stepped back for a wider view and suddenly saw that man as me. I knew what he was begging for: "No more, please, I can't take any more."

I sat down and cried. Brushing paint on the canvas somehow stirred up buried emotions. I couldn't identify what it was in that moment, but I know now what I had touched – a great sadness at all the living I had missed and the emotional cost I paid for my alcoholism.

I accept that some of my wounds from drinking will never fully heal and will drift along with me as a shadow in my heart. I've done a lot of therapy and recovery work and thought I had exhumed most, if not all, of my drinking legacy and come to terms with most of my losses. I discovered otherwise while writing this book when, with my wife's help, I touched some dark unresolved grief. I still grieve the loss of my mother, and that grief has affected how I live. My job now is to understand and honor that grief and bring it fully to light. (see Note 9 for information about grief.)

There's a difference between being healed and being cured. Healing means to make whole again what was damaged; curing means to control or eliminate whatever disrupts the healthy functioning of body, mind, or behavior. These are dictionary definitions, and for addicts like me, the distinction is important.

Healing can take many forms, and different ways work for different people. The goal is the same; just as some people eat meat and others don't, they both share the same goal of getting nourishment.

Curing is a straight-line attempt to control what's wrong, but it seems to me that way doesn't work for someone with an incurable disease. Wounds heal and leave scars.

Why is this important?

It's important because I understand that I drank in part because I couldn't accept that life can be very hard. I was born swaddled in privilege with a silver cradle of promise, and as an adult I believed I was entitled to that birthright as compensation for everything done to me. Drinking, of course, stripped the promise away. I couldn't blame myself for blowing it; instead, I told myself it wasn't my fault. A conspiracy did it.

I've come to understand that living inevitably includes loss; in my case, my mother and niece died and I didn't know how to handle it. I couldn't accept their deaths and move on, and instead wrapped myself in intense anger and frustration. Having a glass of whatever in my hand, or even the anticipation of drinking, quelled those emotions. But the next day, my alcohol defense in neutral, they would flame up inside me again.

In my early AA days, a friend urged me to read The Road Less Traveled by M. Scott Peck. I bought the book, opened to the first line and read this:

"Life is difficult. This is a great truth, one of the greatest truths. It is a great truth because once we truly see this truth, we transcend it. Once that we know that life is difficult -- once we truly understand and accept it – then our life is no longer difficult."

I didn't fully understand those lines at that time, but I did feel comforted.

***

Staying clean and sober is the key to unlocking the hidden doors blocking the path to recovery and sobriety. The first door – willingness to stop using and seek help – is the most important. Many doors that shelter emotional trauma follow, and how many doors one chooses to push open is a personal choice.

My friend Tom D. of the Twelve Step Club walked through the first door into AA and decided to stop there. He's stayed sober for thirty-six years and is just happy to not be drinking. Did that improve his life? Absolutely. Did he change his general attitude towards things? Not so much.

I felt a deep need for more change, so I pushed through more doors, and over the years discovered more about myself. I often choked with fear and denial, but I kept pushing because I wanted more of the emotional sobriety that others had achieved and told me how to reach it.

For me it is a process unfolding. Writing of this book revealed another door I needed to open, behind which lay unresolved grief long buried. As I write this, I'm choosing to step through it. Just being willing to do that has lightened my spirit.

Continuing to grieve and honor my sadness of loss is necessary because too many old habits continue to jump up and bite me. I have to excavate what's driving them.

Francis Weller, a psychotherapist and author who specializes in grief work, shame, and addiction, writes that we can honor and not be ashamed of sadness: "Grief is a powerful solvent, capable of softening the hardest of places in our hearts. Grieving, by its very nature, confirms worth. I am worth crying over: My losses matter."

There are moments when my nose seems pinned against a glass wall blocking me from where I want to go. I don't know what is cementing me in place, but I seek help with a therapist because I can't break through by myself.

Sometimes I feel sad about what I sacrificed to my addiction: not taking my education as far as I could have, hiding in fear of relationships, missing the intellectual ferment, energy, and hope (and yes, the craziness too) of the sixties, and normalcy. I often cry when hearing folk tunes from that time that I heard but never really listened to. I regret not going to Cambridge, beating on my boyhood friends, and the pain I inflicted on my first wife.

I also feel a deep sadness at not having children. But I would have been a terrible father while drinking. I had been sober seventeen years when I first understood how terrible. I moved to Pittsburgh in 2002 to be with Rene and her daughter, Sierra, who was fifteen at the time and endowed with the acute teenage radar for bullshit. Sierra's first impression of me was definitely negative. She was always very polite towards me, and I thought things were going really well until Rene told me that Sierra's politeness was her "kiss of death," i.e., never shall this chasm be bridged. I was surprised to hear that. Politeness was a standard I was raised with as a courtesy to show respect and care for someone. It became clear that Sierra certainly didn't respect me, and I can't blame her for disliking the arrogant and gruff exterior I often showed. I knew that if I wanted Rene in my life, I had to change those attitudes.

I accepted that Sierra would always be Rene's Number One and just let Sierra be however she chose to be around me. That worked. She eventually started to tease me and with a smile call me out on my gruffness and other of my cherished behaviors. I knew then I was in.

Staying sober and working on my emotional flaws helped me develop a loving and trusting relationship with her which has been a huge blessing for me. Sierra embraced me and filled my heart.

One of my greatest losses was any sense of intimacy. I was terrified of being close to anyone at any time, be it male friend or female companion, If I let my guard down, they might find me to be the fraud and failure I knew I was. So, I took hostages, not friends, and I was a terrible sexual partner – I could only engage in sex when I was really drunk, took only what I needed, and never showed interest in my partner's enjoyment. I never gave of myself or shared my fears or feelings with anyone.

Here's what usually happened. I always started a new relationship with a whirlwind of drinking, dining, and dancing. The healthy women soon wanted to slow things down and find out more about me, to look behind my curtain of frenetic partying to see what was really there. I of course always started to back away and keep them at arm's length to protect my secrets.

Frustrated by my triviality and suspecting something was deeply wrong with me, the healthy ones always left to escape the craziness I needed to hide in. The sick ones stuck around, but I'd get bored and toss them aside to find another willing victim. Often in frustration I'd avoid all that and indulge in pornography and masturbation, which was easy, quick, and safe.

For years my wife Rene has told me there's a deep sorrow inside me that I've been unable or unwilling to touch. I used to dismiss that notion because I am rarely sad. But the truth is, I'm also rarely really, unabashedly happy. I started looking inside again as I was writing this book, and to my surprise some patterns became clear.

I don't wear loud clothes – Hawaiian shirts excepted, although with some unease. I'll see a really colorful shirt, one splashed with reds and greens and purples, the whole palette, and I think, Man, that would look great on me! For a second or two, I'd see myself strutting down some busy street like Kramer, of "Seinfeld" fame, in the Technicolor Dreamcoat. But I back up -- no, it's too daring, too revealing. My wardrobe consists of blue jeans and dark, earth-tone shirts and pullovers. No sparkles there (that's gonna change now, though).

My heart breaks when I see baby birds begging their mothers for food; their wings spread wide, body lowered, beak extended, making a beseeching bird call. I know intellectually that mothers are trying to wean their kids off of parent-provided food, but my heart breaks when I see or hear it. When Rene and I lived in Pittsburgh, I tore down a wire fence in the backyard so a baby robin could flutter to its mother calling for it to come.

I also uncovered sadness for a loss I never expected—the

emotional boost drinking gave me, until the end of my drunkenness. Don't get me wrong, I'm thrilled to be sober and experience few gray days. I certainly don't miss the terrible desolation, the awful hangovers, the harm I caused, the stupid shit I pulled, the dread of what could have happened on any given blacked-out night. But there are times I miss the camaraderie, the romance of cocktailing and the rituals adorning wine, and especially being in the center and important in a group. I'm often reminded of just how powerful those drinking rituals were for me, especially now, short of churchgoing, when I feel a lack of ritual in my life. Reading books and walking in the woods fill me with joy, but they lack the jazz and whiz-bang that for two decades fed my constant need for excitement that seemed ever harder to reach. I still feel the pull of it even after being sober for thirty-five years. I don't think of it as a defect, but rather as a reminder that I am an addict. And that I'm okay.

My wife and I sometimes join friends for a dinner out, and I watch as they each order a glass of wine and feel a sadness when asking for mineral water. I cover myself by telling the waiter that I'm the driver. As the evening progresses, I sense in them – deeply, and with some sadness -- the well-being I often felt when toasting a first or second drink with my buddies.

As the evening progresses, I notice that their postures ease, conversations deepen, laughter rises with blossoming intimacy. I'm always part of the talking, but sometimes I feel that old, old sense of being left out of the secret, of being on the outside looking in.

Today I know that feeling is what's called "euphoric recall," a pining for the good old days while forgetting the bad old days. Many of us in recovery experience that, and when I do, I chuckle to myself: I'm an alcoholic, why would I be any different? And it goes away, only to rise up again. I don't expect that euphoric recall will ever disappear, and I accept that. My daily task is to take spiritual care of myself, help others, and remember where I used to be.

I found these comforting quotes online. "Grief, by definition, will never fully 'go away,' because it is the force that drives your 'becoming' after the loss of something. It is not an emotion experienced at this moment, but part of your new life." And this from ghostwriter and editor Kate Ward: "If love is the song of our lives, then grief is the echo. It is the result of loving things outside ourselves – as we were meant to – and then losing them" (Quota.com/How-do-sadness-and-grief-differ).

The most difficult stuff I've had to deal with is more spiritual than physical. The Twelve Steps of AA helped me understand that the world doesn't revolve around me. I worked to change myself so I could stand in this world as an honest, responsible, grateful and forgiving man. To do that I had to grow up, accept my past, change my thinking, and honor my sadness.

To repeat, AA meetings are not therapy sessions. The Twelve Steps don't touch on grief. They focus on what we did, not so much on why we did it – that's assumed because we're alcoholics. Drinking is the major reason, but there's more. Bill Wilson, a founder of AA, came to understand when he was twenty-one years sober that deeper work is needed to achieve what he termed, "emotional sobriety" and "Stage II recovery." He concluded that we need to probe more deeply into why we still act as we always have. (See Note 10 to read Wilson's letter.)

What's next for me about grief? Accepting that I have it, that the sadness I've described will always occupy a place in my heart. I will probably cry many more cleansing tears. Just knowing and accepting that sadness lies there frees me to live joyously without fear.

I can tell you this, though: If something like the sixties comes around again, I'll jump in to partake of the energy, change, and joy of those days.

CHAPTER 14
GRATITUDE

Traits don't change, states of mind do.
--Elizabeth Strout

It takes courage to grow up and become who you really are.
--e.e. cummings

I will always remember Bill. He was an AA Old Timer with a gazillion years of sobriety who walked cane in hand into the Twelve Step Club several times a week. He sat down in the same chair in the same meeting every time. I didn't like him at first because he seemed to be a retired working man, a shot-and-beer-joint drinker, and, hey! I could have gone to Cambridge!

Bill was as reliable as night follows day. No matter the topic he always said the same thing: "You gotta cultivate an attitude of gratitude." No more, no less. I'd look at him and think: "I'm supposed to be grateful to be sitting in these stupid meetings and listening to these fools?"

That was my attitude then, and it's pretty typical for newcomers. Those new to meetings move into a different world where people speak an alien language about happiness and gratitude. My first reaction was to dismiss what I didn't understand as just so much bullshit.

Many, like me, were never taught about gratitude. We were raised to be satisfied with "success," which meant following rules and meeting expectations. *Happiness* had nothing to do with it. *Grateful?* As a kid I often heard grownups tell me to be grateful for my food, even if I didn't like it. Those "starving kids in China" were no incentive for me to eat those stone-cold peas.

I didn't know how to be grateful; that's something I had to learn. I didn't know how to look on the bright side of things, because I had been blinded by dark thinking for so long. My code was, "Do unto others before they can do it unto me." I lived with a mindset of scarcity, blinded to opportunities and promise. My glass was always half empty, and I had to learn how to see it half full. That started to shift when I began to try out some good advice: "Fake it 'til you make it." Just go through the motions, they said, and be surprised at what happens.

Tom and Nona suggested I start small by thinking of one thing I did well in a day. Do a kindness for someone, they said; for example, carry a heavy grocery bag for an elderly woman out to her car. I started washing the coffee cups after a meeting. They also said to show respect by trying to take in what someone said, and to mentally say "thank you" to someone. Doing these things changed my brain chemistry and, amazingly, I started to feel some twinges of happiness.

There's actual science behind this. A publication on gratitude by The Harvard Medical School states: "Gratitude is scientifically proven to take the focus away from your struggles, shortcomings and misfortunes, and redirect them to the goodness in your life." Practicing gratitude is also connected to good health and greater energy and vitality, to say nothing of increasing your happiness.

Gratitude has also proven to help sex abuse victims begin to live full lives. Rachel Warth, author of *Sex Abuse Victim Gratitude Journal: A Journey of Self-healing after Sexual Violation, Molestation or Rape*, says this: "Starting a day with gratitude will not cancel or erase the past, but it can help you own your day, own your life as you move forward."

How does this relate to the 12 Steps? The answer was obvious. I had to break my armor and open my mind to the idea that I could change and open my heart to gratitude, that there might be some hope for me after all.

***

So now you have some idea of my background, upbringing, and history as a recovering alcoholic. I've tried to adequately describe how I changed from being a desperate, almost suicidal drunk to the sober man I am today. It took a miracle, hard work, determination and, yes, some luck for that to happen. I wouldn't be sober today without the friends I found in AA and my neighbors in whom I found trust and love. They told me the truth about me (something I usually didn't want to hear), and this gave me the courage to finally disinter my secrets, get honest, and change my behavior.

It took a while, but I came to realize how much at ease I felt with them, and how similar I was in background and character to everyone else in AA. I became willing to work with my sponsor Ron who patiently listened to my complaints and often told me, "Get off the cross, we need the wood." I sought therapy when I needed help. I became willing, finally, to work the 12 Steps as best I could.

Doing so, I learned to honor myself and give others their due. And I learned to accept that I don't have to be perfect to live the life I want. I had to honor the fear, pain, and love in my core, and flush the bullshit. I came to know how exhilarating it feels to be honest about everything. I didn't have to bob and weave anymore and could dance to my own music.

CHAPTER 15
NATURE'S BLESSING

Keep close to nature's heart... and break clear away,
once in a while...wash your spirit clean.
--John Muir

I wrote in my Step-Three discussion about taking my first trip sober to Monument Valley and Arizona and how that place changed me. More amazement awaited me in the Grand Canyon a few years later.

It was late summer 1995 and near the end of my Flagstaff life. I had lived there for four plus years and worked construction four days a week. The other three days you would usually find me on a Grand Canyon trail, or back in Monument Valley, or hiking in one of the national parks in southern Utah.

I fell in love with that landscape. I craved hiking along narrow and winding sculptured slot canyon trails in silence so deep I could hear blood coursing through my ears. I negotiated open-air tricky trails under skies of the deepest azure blue. I scrambled over ancient sand dune slick rock, and rested in the shade of junipers to feel a whispering breeze. I couldn't get enough of it. Now I knew I was at one with this place. That sculpted, earth-colored land filled a spiritual hole left in me from my heartbreak when I was a kid. I thirsted for more, like a parched nomad seeking an oasis.

In late July, I was soon to leave for graduate school at the University of Illinois in Champaign-Urbana. I needed to say goodbye to my favorite place, the Grand Canyon, and decided to do one last solo hike. I drove to the Thunder River trailhead on the North Rim. My truck was the only vehicle there, which thrilled me -- I would be alone in the canyon with no one else around, surrounded by silence, just the way I liked it.

The trail starts at an elevation of 7,200 feet with a steep descent of about 800 feet to the Esplanade, a unique formation in the canyon. Hikers typically camp there for a night and cache water for the climb back up.

The Thunder River trail, like all the canyon trails, was laid out to intersect places where the Red Wall, an 800-foot vertical layer of very hard red sandstone, is degraded enough for a hiker to descend into Surprise Valley, which is at 3600 feet. Thunder River, by the way, is one of the world's shortest rivers; it drops 1,200 feet in a half mile, making it the steepest river in the United States. It joins Tapeats Creek, which flows to the Colorado River at 1950 feet.

I slept a bit uneasily that night, the old fears gnawing at me as I scrunched in my sleeping bag and kept a wary eye. By morning the weather had changed to gathering clouds promising rain -- not a surprise since July is the beginning of the annual monsoon season.

A typical day at that time of year dawns with a clear sky. A few clouds appear mid-morning and grow into small thunderstorms with gusts of showers, all to dissipate in a clear sky by evening. This particular morning, clouds formed early into high piles that majestically floated above the canyon's crags and gullies, dressed with rising crowns laced with lightning and thunder.

I packed light, because I learned on my first canyon hike that every pound weighs a ton on weary legs plodding up a trail. Out of respect for the place you must hump out every ounce you hauled in – minus what you've eaten. But I packed a bit light this time. I had a plastic ground cloth, pad, sleeping bag, some dehydrated food with a plastic bowl and spoon, a backpacking stove, a water filter and a gallon of water for the descent and one to cache. About thirty-five pounds total, but no rain gear.

I hiked the mile or so to the Red Wall descent and sat there for about an hour trying to decide if I should climb down and stay wet or turn around and beat the rain. I chose the dry route and retraced my steps back to my water cache. I left one behind for anyone in need of water, which is a courtesy shared by most hikers. The weather was changing quickly, and as I started hiking up a talus slope before the steep wall, a nearby small thunderstorm started to throw out horizontal lightning flashes. That made hiking up the wall pretty dangerous and I decided not to push my luck. I sat in a ravine to watch and wait.

Spread wide before me was a vast expanse about twelve miles wide where the canyon bends to the south. I watched entranced as several small thunderheads floated across that vast space and counted the seconds between the lightning flashes and rumbling echoes.

I sat there for I don't know how long awestruck by the beauty and immensity of what was before me. It was the most beautiful thing I had ever seen. And then I had an epiphany -- I knew deep down that I could die that very moment and it wouldn't make a damn bit of difference to anything there. I remembered what Catholic theologian Belden C. Lane had written in a Christian Century magazine article, "Fierce Landscapes and the Indifference of God": We are saved in the end by the things that ignore us. (The full article is available online.)

For the very first time – I was then ten years sober -- I understood what he meant and felt truly in the presence of a Power greater than myself. Nothing mattered more than that I was in that place and part of its majesty. I felt a well-being like others had described that I had searched for. I cried.

My mind blew open. I had always thought that I would be humiliated to be reduced to nothing, but instead I felt exalted and blessed. Some might say I had a religious experience in the canyon, that God's grace found me there. Maybe. What I do know for certain is I experienced a profound awakening I can hardly describe that revealed the most important things in my life – loving and accepting love, friends, kindness to everyone and everything, and awe for the beauty that surrounds me wherever I am. I was shaken alive just like I was on the day when I knew I had to quit drinking. Each was a special moment that saved and changed me.

Sometime later I shouldered my pack and started up the trail. I got in my truck and headed back to Flagstaff feeling in my gut that my world had changed forever. That exaltation stayed with me until I hit graduate school.

It was then that the world crashed in on me again, consuming my energy and attention. I was starting a new career in journalism and learning how to navigate the pressure and deadlines of a newsroom. To keep my priorities in order, I tried to feel the peace of my experience in the canyon. I could spend a hectic week filing under deadline several stories for the front page of a newspaper, and on my days off drive to the mountains or to a park to hike, listen, and refresh my spirit.

No two experiences like these can ever be the same, so however it's achieved, spiritual awakening blesses all of us in the same way by endowing us with the freedom to choose who we will be and what we want. "Freedom" to choose is a key one. I learned that my life is my choice.

I want to share a message I learned from my experiences in nature. I feel very privileged to be among the few who could hike into the Grand Canyon and other amazing places, but don't let my good fortune discourage you from seeking your own spiritual awakening anywhere in the natural world, including your own back yard by a tree.

I've spent time in state forests in Pennsylvania, city parks in Washington state, and walked along rivers in different cities, and in every case, I have felt the beauty and power of nature. It's available to anyone. I learned to take the time to rest and watch the sun rise over a lake or listen to birds sing and wind whisper in trees in a city park. Doing this simple thing always opens my heart no matter where I am.

I'm fascinated with trees. They're amazing creatures with much to teach us. I often stop on a trail to look at how a tree has adapted to its environment. It's an ancient story. A seed drops to the ground and takes root. Some seeds fall on old stumps, take root, and in time grow roots down along the sides and around. The roots thicken as the stump wastes away giving strength and support for the trunk. Some look like an octopus standing on its arms, still straight and reaching for the sun. A forest shows any number of variations of this—trees are immensely creative. For example, a seed falls on a rock ledge and germinates in the moss or any bit of soil around. The seedling knows it's in an iffy situation and sends tendrils in several directions. Some older trees create huge roots that use cracks or stretch behind for a strong grip. Sometimes a tree grows right next to it and both cling to the edge and intertwine, almost like an embrace, for mutual support.

Here's my point: trees show how recovery works. They do what it takes to survive and grow. They seek help when needed. They dig deep for sustenance and reach for the sky.

CHAPTER 16
THE UNEXPECTED GIFT

*Sometimes life drops blessings in your lap without you
lifting a finger. Serendipity, they call it.*
--Charlton Heston

That word "serendipity" is one of my favorites because of its definition: "The art of finding good things unlooked for." I've added a few words of my own to that: "Always expect the unexpected. Life happens with ups and downs, but staying hopeful makes the 'art.'"

I used to think that serendipity was for others, but a surprising event in early October 2001 proved me wrong. Being sober is what made the following story possible.

On the seventh day of that month, I opened a letter from Rene and almost passed out. Hearing from her was a million-to-one shot I never expected, and it hit me like a ton of bricks that forever, once again, changed my life.

I first met Rene in freshman year in high school and thought her the most beautiful girl I had ever seen (and still do). Rene was dating Fred, the captain of the football and wrestling teams. I desperately wanted to play varsity football, figuring I would beat the hell out of Fred on the field and earn the chance to be with her. Without the gridiron I felt totally outclassed, but Dad refused to let me play. I felt emasculated when he told me no, and I begged. And begged more, only to hear the same answer. I hated him for not letting me do what I so desperately wanted to do. Today I'm immensely grateful for not playing, and I thank Dad for keeping me in the stable. As screwed up and full of anger as I was, I probably would have severely injured myself on the field and maybe damaged another player. And today I can still walk and bend over without pain and usually remember where I left the car keys.

I had already been drinking for a few years and my self-confidence had flatlined, so I didn't know how to ask Rene for a date. I did walk her home a few times, maybe even caried her books. One day I screwed up my courage and asked her out, and to my surprise, she said yes. It was junior year. I had my driver's license, and all I needed was a car.

My Grandmother Norma said I could drive her car, but at the last minute she changed her mind. I pleaded with Dad to let me drive the Buick 225, but he refused. Instead, to my acute embarrassment, he said he would drive us to the movie theater and pick us up.

I hated him even more for not letting me use the car. In my mind he was only confirming my worthlessness. Rene tells me that it didn't bother her at the time. At the World's Fair in 1964 I bought her a jade necklace that she still has.

We went off to college. I went to Carleton and she entered the University of Wisconsin in Madison. Somehow (neither of us can remember how) we made contact with each other in the Spring of 1970. I was soon to graduate, and Rene was student teaching in Bloomington, Minnesota. We met for lunch and I asked her out, and -- surprise! -- she told me she was getting married in June.

For some bizarre reason, I did what I thought was the gentlemanly thing and attended her wedding. I left a card with my best wishes at the church (she still has it today). After the "I dos," I slipped out of the church and walked home. Weird.

I knew then she was gone for good, and I pushed her out of my mind, but sometimes an oldies station would play "Don't walk away Renee," and there she'd be.

Thirty-one years later in late August 2001, I was living in Arlington, Texas, and working as a reporter in a bureau of the Dallas

Morning News. I had been dating a woman in Fort Worth for a couple of months, more or less to have something to do outside the office. My role in that "relationship" was to provide the meal and movie ticket, which attracted lukewarm attention from her, and cooled any real interest in me. I had mired myself in a dating rut.

One Sunday morning I lay in bed feeling a bit disgusted with myself. I had spent another Saturday night with that woman trying out a new restaurant. As always, I paid the bill and flat-footed my inept way through line dancing lessons. I just couldn't get my feet to go with the beat, which made the evening even more boring. I mulled all that over and finally made a promise to myself: "I don't care if I'm celibate the rest of my life, but I'm never doing that again." I closed that cell allowing another door to open. It took only a few weeks for that to happen.

I wasn't holding myself in reserve for the right woman, I wanted out of the dating rut I had fallen into. I wanted a partner to adventure with who also loved music, books, hikes in woods and traveling. And amazingly, she soon arrived.

In September 2001, I spent a week in Arizona taking care of Dad, who was suffering from Parkinson's disease, to give his wife, Mary, a break to see her grandchildren. I flew back home to Texas to a full mailbox. I pulled out a textured envelope with Rene's name on the return address. I thought how strange that a business would have the same name as Rene's. Curious, I opened it.

I read, "Dear Bob," and almost passed out. It was a bolt out of the blue, a million-to-one shot that gave me the second greatest shock of my life (the first shock knocked me awake in that phone booth).

I learned in that instant to expect the unexpected. As of this writing, we've been together almost twenty years and married for ten. A couple months later, we fell in love.

Rene's letter had arrived when I was about to move to Durango, Colorado, for a reporting job with The Durango Herald. Rene was living in Pittsburgh with her daughter Sierra. I knew in my heart that she was the One, but I also loved being a journalist in a Colorado mountain town.

I knew the decision I had to make was a big one. Stay near the mountains I loved or risk everything by moving to Steel Town without a guarantee that this relationship would work. I decided to trust the unexpected, listened to my gut -- my Truth Speaker -- and took the leap for love. But I moved to Pittsburgh with a big problem. I didn't know how to be in a committed relationship. I had never committed to anyone for more than a few months; commitment to any person took a back seat to drinking. Commitment was an alien concept to a guy like me. I was like a flat stone skipping along the surface and never going deep.

Rene nearly ditched me a few times for my negativity, which was my default place in my fear of vulnerability and intimacy. I could hear the thin ice cracking at times and had another decision to make. If I really wanted her in my life, I had to change how I thought and acted. To me our relationship was a still rough gemstone, and I had no idea how hard the polishing would be.

How hard soon became clear. I first had to give up my old ways, especially the flashes of anger when things weren't going as I wanted. I remembered that my MO in previous relationships was to blame the woman for whatever wasn't working right and use that to justify my leaving before they tossed me out. I know now that it was all about my abandonment issues, which I worked through by trusting that Rene and I were okay.

After a few spats – Rene is a very strong-willed feminist and wouldn't put up with my stuff -- I realized I had to change how I responded to her criticisms and complaints. My old way was to yell back and claim unfairness, but I knew that wasn't going to work with her. I changed by keeping my mouth shut and listening to what she was saying. I made a rule that no matter what she said or how angry I might be, I would not respond for a while. This helped me to cool down and think clearly about whether what she has said was true about me and how much of it was about her own stuff. Then we could talk calmly and get down to what was really going on. It still works for both of us.

Keeping my mouth shut was hard. I missed my old way of talking louder and longer than the other guy to establish my dominance, and I had to change that. It became much easier once I accepted that we're both stubborn individualists and occasional fireworks will flare up. But even in the heat of an argument we both our deep love for each other as non-negotiable.

CHAPTER 17
MY OWN WORK GOES ON

What lies behind us and what lies before us are tiny matters compared to what lies within us.
--Ralph Waldo Emerson

All that is gold does not glitter.
--J.R.R. Tolkien

When I first quit drinking, I never expected that life would be so topsy-turvy. AA friends told me that sobriety is a great upheaval and would upend everything I had taken for granted. Getting sober helped me look back and deal with my past, and with time, I could sense how I'd changed and honestly see what hadn't changed about me. Living sober is like peeling an onion, the deeper you go, the more you see.

I write this now thirty-five years sober, and yes, I still have work to do. I say that not in frustration but out of acceptance. I'll never be perfect and don't have to be, and life problems will probably resurrect old behaviors I thought I'd laid to rest. My life now is one surprise after another. I glory in the good surprises – those are easy and fun -- and tackle the unwelcome ones as best I can. Life happens and accepting that reality enriches my sobriety.

Here are some issues that I'm working on.

I'm a natural born isolator, and when Rene's gone camping for a few days, I tend to close the door and stay inside. On my first day alone, I usually feel lonely and uncomfortable, but I get used to it as the days pass. After all, I spent most of my life feeling alone. When she walks back in a few days later, I sometimes (silently) think, "What are you doing here?" More work to do here, for sure.

At times when alone, I look to chocolate ice cream to cure my loneliness, but that never works, even though I always think it might. The real cure is to get off the couch, turn off the TV or computer and go outside the house for a walk or to a meeting. Doing that helps me to feel much better.

The 12 Step Club, my first AA meeting place, kept a rack of candy bars at the coffee bar to help newcomers stave off cravings. Alcohol is absorbed in the blood through the stomach wall, and it used to satisfy the sugar craving that sprouted in me as a child. I drank so much alcohol that I rarely ate dessert, but as soon as I quit drinking, zoooom! I couldn't get enough candy bars, donuts, ice cream, cake, pie, you name it. I rarely crave alcohol, but sugar is a different story.

Today I still eat sugar even though I know it's not good for my health. I perform the perfect addict's dance around this substance – I bargain, swear off, promise myself to never touch it again, feel shame after inhaling it, but so far, I have been unwilling to quit. I'm as delusional about sugar as I was alcohol, and I use sugar to relieve something in me that I haven't identified yet. To be honest, I haven't marshaled the courage to end it.

I speak about this often at meetings, almost always to know-ing chuckles. But for me the bottom-line issue is: I know it's ad-dictive thinking. I'm working on it...some of the time.

I hate routine, love learning new things, often look for adven-ture in forests and canyons, and am a bit scatterbrained to boot. All true. My wife Rene's biggest complaint is that I don't always pay attention and listen well. I often mishear or disregard things she says and often forget what she said or what I heard. I'm better than when we started working on this issue, because I'm learning to focus on what's at hand, stop hurrying, be more patient, judge less and meditate more.

One other really important thing. This goes way back to my toddlerhood and what I learned from my sister catering to my every need. I came to believe that someone would always provide for my needs and clean up after my failings. And if they didn't, they weren't worthy of my lordly attention and I'd tell them to go to hell. I still carry that self-absorption around.

I recently came to understand what that really meant. Rene has repeatedly pointed out that I was too absorbed in myself and unaware of others, and often didn't do what I needed to do for myself. For example, when hiking on a chilly day, my sinuses run and my right eye tears, but I never thought to bring tissues with me. I always asked Rene if she had some. A minor issue, you might think, but a symptom of my underlying assumption that someone would make sure I always had what I needed.

This issue is now on the surface and I'm working to make sure to stay responsible for my own needs and wants. I take my own tissues when we hike, and I try to be completely present when we talk. I'm working on slowing down, both in thinking and acting, to hear the important stuff the first time.

***

Rene and I worked as camp hosts for two summers, and boy, did my dark habits spill out in spades. Over the years I've been critical and somewhat dismissive of service workers; my gruffness becomes obvious in stores and restaurants where I demand respectful, prompt, and precise attention. Rene has often criticized me for that. I usually brushed it off, until the last weeks of a difficult, hot, very busy summer hosting a large campground.

The campground is a hot spot for boaters and partiers, not the usual types I'm used to hanging out with. What emerged in me was some really old stuff.

Most of the campers were really nice people and a pleasure to be in the woods with. But others, a minority for sure, seemed to not give a damn about anything but themselves and their own pleasure. (Sounds just like me back in the day.)

Many of them flaunted the campground rules prohibiting the consumption of alcohol and pot, which they had agreed to follow when making their reservations. They created most of the drinking and noise problems we had to deal with. Many of them left their campsites strewn with trash. We camp hosts were not allowed to enforce the no-drinking rule, so our bosses had the honor of kicking several individuals out for drunkenness.

I often ranted about those lousy, ignorant, show-off campers and wanted to wreak vengeance upon them with hellfire and brimstone. How dare they violate the pristine silence of my precious trees! Rene reminded me that a positive attitude and showing them some respect was the better way to set things right. And she assured me I would feel better as a result.

But I realized that I needed them to respect me as host and follow the campground rules I was hired to enforce, and when they ignored those rules I vaulted back to the high moral plane where I could glare down and judge them for their sins. I had fallen right back to my teen years and my need for self-justification. Finally, I admitted that "my way or the highway" wouldn't work and worked hard to keep calm about it all. Rene was right – I did feel better for it.

I'm working on this, too.

CHAPTER 18
LIFE IS GREAT

Be thankful for what you have, you'll end up having more. If you concentrate on what you don't have, you will never have enough.
--Oprah Winfrey

I want to close with the promise folks told me when I first sobered up. If I worked diligently to be honest about myself and responsible for my thinking and behavior, then my life, health, and mind would change in ways unimaginable and all to the good.

For me, such extensive change required all the diligence and perseverance I could muster, plus a lot of time, self-patience, and often hard, painful work. And as you've read, I still need to do even more work.

Where's my sobriety leading me? I have no destination, but I know that working to better myself will deepen the abundance I now enjoy. As much as I've changed, I'm eager for more changes to come.

To help that along, I still attend AA meetings, though not nearly as many as I used to, to stay in touch with fellow alcoholics and addicts. I need to hear their stories and struggles to remind myself who I used to be. I will always be an alcoholic, and sobriety is an ongoing and ever-deepening process. Accepting that as a fact makes my life so much better.

The Twelve Promises listed below are the "magic" that my sponsor Ron urged me to wait for. They are the reward I've been given for doing the work to achieve emotional and long-term sobriety. They are named The Promises because they come true for anyone willing to leap into abstinence and work to change themselves. Julia Cameron put it this way in The Artis's Way : "Leap, and the net will appear." I took that leap thirty-five years ago, the support I needed appeared, and my path to sobriety unfolded before me.

I read these promises as a daily blessing:

The Twelve Promises

We are going to know a new freedom and a new happiness.

We will not regret the past nor wish to shut the door on it.

We will comprehend the word serenity, and we will know peace.

No matter how far down the scale we have gone, we will see how our experience can benefit others.

That feeling of uselessness and self-pity will disappear.

We will lose interest in selfish things and gain interest in our fellows.

Self-seeking will slip away.

Our whole attitude and outlook on life will change.

Fear of people and of economic insecurity will leave us.

We will intuitively know how to handle situations which used to baffle us.

We will suddenly realize that God is doing for us what we could not do for ourselves.

Are these extravagant promises? We think not.

They are being fulfilled among us, sometimes quickly, sometimes slowly.

They will always materialize if we work for them.

Final Thoughts

My greatest blessing with emotional sobriety is serenity. Serenity for me is not a permanent mental condition. I have to cultivate it every day, just as I do with gratitude and humility. I do so with music or words when my happiness fades into the shadows. On such days I try to remember a verse John Stewart, a former member of the Kingston Trio, wrote in one of my favorite songs: "Those aren't clouds on the horizon, they're the shadows of the angel's wings."

I use this lyric to reaffirm that a silver lining rises from the heart of every cloud which tells me that I can deal with just about anything as long as I stay sober.

I decided to publish this story in the hope that it might help someone who is struggling to stay abstinent from addiction. If my story helps just one person do that, I will be very happy.

It is my hope that publishing this book might help you or someone you love.

***

NOTES

1. Alcoholics Anonymous (Page 12)

AA is an international "mutual aid" fellowship whose only requirement for membership "is a desire to quit drinking." In 2016 AA had nearly two million members worldwide.

It was founded in 1935 in Akron, Ohio, by Bill Wilson and Dr. Bob Smith, who met and talked about their drinking and struggles to stay sober. They also talked about solutions, which with help from other early members, became the AA Bible: Alcoholics Anonymous: The Story of How More Than One Hundred Men Have Recovered from Alcoholism written in 1939. That title became the name of the organization and is now referred to as "The Big Book."

The Big Book sets forth the AA program in the Twelve Steps and includes the Twelve Traditions, which urges members to remain anonymous in public media, and refrain from discussing "outside issues" during meetings. The Traditions also require AA groups to accept only voluntary member contributions and not accept "outside" donations. The purpose of the Traditions is to keep groups and members focused on AA's sole purpose, which is "To help other alcoholics achieve sobriety."

The AA Twelve Steps have been adapted to many other mutual help addiction recovery programs including Narcotics Anonymous, Gamblers Anonymous, Codependents Anonymous and Sex Addicts Anonymous.

2. Secular Recovery Groups (Page 12)

Alcoholics Anonymous calls on people to turn their "wills and their lives" over to a higher power and find a spiritual awakening. That continues to work for me, although I detested the hand-holding and saying the Lord's Prayer at the end of my very first meeting. Most people I've found feel pretty much the same – some like me stick around, and others search for alternatives.

Most alternatives are more secular, are free to join for those willing to follow the main requirement for membership: achieve and maintain abstinence. Here are a few:

• Self-Management and Recovery Training (SMART) – smartrecovery.org The SMART welcomes anyone suffering any addiction. Its focus is on obtaining and maintaining motivation, learning to manage urges, handling emotions, thoughts and behaviors, all to find and strike a balance in life.

• Women For Sobriety – womenforsobriety.org

This group's doctrine is that behaviors follow thoughts, and changing thoughts can alter behaviors. It also encourages women to love themselves, exercise control and potentially experience spiritual growth.

• LifeRing Secular Recovery – lifering.org

Each person has the power within themselves to control addiction, and every addict has an "Addict Self" and a 'Sober Self." This group does not rely on a "higher power," sponsors or certain steps to attain sobriety, but asks that each person find strength and control within themselves.

• Moderation Management – moderation.org

This group does not require abstinence, but invites people to join who sense alcohol is a rising issue in their lives. Its meetings focus on finding balance in life and changing negative behaviors into healthier and more positive ones.

3. Sobriety Success

Another issue difficult to address is: How successful is AA in helping people achieve long term sobriety? Are there other programs available that do better? The answer: it depends on who's talking.

The Big Book claims that 50 percent achieve long-term sobriety, but addiction specialists in various studies derive an AA success rate at 8 to 12 percent. The issue involves definitions: what exactly is meant by "sobriety?" or "long term?" Is it defined as total abstinence over a period of years as defined by AA, or reduction of frequency of drinking and alcohol-related problems over several months as claimed by the SMART Recovery online program?

The 2014 National Survey on Drug Use and Health found that about 20 million adults aged 12 and above struggle with "substance abuse disorder."

Some recovery programs were created by folks turned off by the religious connotations in AA, which calls for finding and believing in a high power, God if you choose, as a vehicle for recovery. LifeRing Secular Recovery is one, SMART Recovery is another that focus members on finding inside themselves a definition and determination to moderate or abstain from using. Many rely on scientific studies of the role of psychotherapy or neurotherapy in treating symptoms, but several, including SMART, borrow from AA the idea of community support through meetings either online or in person.

Each of these programs show some success, but all run into

what Dr. Freidman wrote: "Addiction is one of the most puzzling and fascinating human behaviors, one that reflects a complex interplay among genes, biology, psychology and environment."

4. The Addict Brain

Here are some facts on how addiction affects the brain. Some discussions of these are quite technical, but research has described the physical, emotional ,and mental consequences of active addiction.

You can read these in more detail at the following sites or conduct an internet search:

From "Buzzed, The Straight facts about the most used and abused drugs from Alcohol and Ecstasy" 2014, Cynthia Kuhn et.al.

"Never Enough, The Neuroscience and Experience of Addiction," Judith Grisel, 2019.

Specifics for alcohol use:

a. Alcohol affects two types of neuronal transmitters which depress brain activity and inhibit formation of new memories. That explains why, after an extended bout of drinking, it can be difficult to remember all of what happened. In some cases, extreme drinking can blot out entire chunks of time with no memory, i.e., so-called blackouts. Alcohol is classified as a "sedative-hypnotic."

b. Alcohol drinking increases the release of dopamine, the main chemical messenger in the reward centers of the brain. The first minutes of drinking activates the pleasure circuits of the brain, a so-called "dopamine rush" which disappears after the alcohol level stops rising. That can result in "chasing the high," i.e., motivating the drinker to consume more alcohol to keep the pleasure feelings going.

c. How much can you drink before causing health problems? Most studies show that very moderate drinking brings some health benefits, but two drinks a day as an average can significantly increase the risk of dying from heart disease or cancer. Excessive, chronic drinking leads to stroke and heart disease; high blood pressure; liver problems, including steatosis (fatty liver), alcohol hepatitis, fibrosis and cirrhosis; pancreatitis; and increased risk of various cancers including mouth, esophagus, larynx, breast, liver colon and rectum.

    a. Brain imaging techniques show that long-term alcohol use causes shrinkage in some areas of the brain. Those who stop drinking and remain abstinent will experience recovery of brain tissue.

    b. Other brain imaging studies suggest drug addicts and alcoholics have fewer dopamine receptors in the brain's reward pathway than do non-addicts. "Addicts may simply have a lower baseline of happiness than other people," wrote Richard A. Friedman in a May 5, 2014 New York Times review of "The Sober Truth." The authors of that book argued their view of the ineffectiveness of 12 Step Programs.

There are five areas of mental ability that are compromised by chronic alcohol abuse: memory formation, abstract thinking problem solving, attention and concentration, and perception of emotion. As many as 70 percent of those seeking treatment for alcohol-related problems suffer significant impairment of these abilities. Those heavy drinkers who quit partially recover these functions in the first or second month, but most never fully recover these functions even after years of abstinence. "It is reasonable to estimate that people who drink three or more drinks per day on average are at substantial risk of developing permanent deficits in certain cognitive abilities... Three drinks per day appears, from the research, to be something of a threshold.

One of the main risk factors for alcohol addiction is drinking to self-medicate, to block out emotional or social problems. Research is inconclusive on the extent of genetic factors, but "It is very clear [however] that alcoholism, like diabetes, runs in families. With no family history of alcoholism, the risk of developing alcohol abuse problems is about 10 percent for men and 5 percent for women. However, the risk nearly doubles if there is a family history of alcohol problems.

Women who drink are at significantly greater risk for liver damage than men, even if they drink less alcohol or drink for a shorter period of time. Women are also at greater risk for developing pancreas and high blood pressure problems than men; drinking also increases the risk for breast cancer.

The above are just some snippets of a large and growing field of scientific studies, and there are numerous online sources and books available for more detailed information.

5. Reasons People Use (Page 7)

The following information can be found at Recoveryintune.com. Many people begin experimenting with drugs or alcohol in response to peer pressure, curiosity, or to cope with daily stress, mental illness or a history of trauma. But not everyone who abuses drugs and alcohol will go to the level of addiction or use disorder. The US National Library of Medicine estimates 18 million people in the United States suffer from some kind of alcohol use disorder. There is no way to predict a person's use habits will develop into an addiction, but there are specific factors that are recognized as contributing to a person's predilection for addiction.

• Having a close relative, especially a parent or sibling, with substance abuse issues. Psych Central estimates 28 million children have an alcoholic parent.
• Being diagnosed with a mental health condition such as anxiety, major depression, bipolar disorder, PTSD, etc.
• Having a history of childhood trauma such as poverty, discrimination, neglect and physical and psychological abuse.
• Having early exposure, meaning the earlier a person begins using alcohol or drugs, the greater potential for addiction to develop (I started drinking at 12, which seems a fairly common age for most men in AA).
• A history of childhood aggressiveness, violence, or poor social skills.
• Inadequate parental supervision in childhood history.
• General availability of and access to intoxicating substances.

Addiction inflicts several emotional and physical side effects. Among these are:

• Mood swings, depression, irritability, agitation, and aggression.
• Intense cravings
• Resorting to substance abuse as a means to cope with stress or unwanted thoughts or feelings
• Continuing to believe one's substance abuse is "normal" and not problematic despite adverse consequences such as

financial and legal issues, tense relationships, poor academic performance or loss of employment.
• Becoming defensive when confronted about substance abuse
• Experiencing periods of fatigue and lack of motivation
• Unexplainable episodes of high anxiety, intense fear, and paranoia
• Attempts to quit often followed by relapses.

For parents and loved ones, here are some red flags to look for:

• Abrupt and radical changes in mood or personality in combination with known drug and alcohol use.
• Unusual deception and secretiveness.
• Association with a new and possibly sketchy social circle that appears to glorify and engage in substance abuse.
• Frequent examples of significant problems with family, friends, coworkers and peers that didn't appear before.

6. Genetics

An international group of more than 100 scientists created an extensive database to collect information on smoking and alcohol abuse behaviors. Nature and nurture is a phrase describing research that shows a person's health is a result of the dynamics between genes and the environment. The National Institute on Drug Abuse reported the scientists measured behaviors including the age when smoking started and ended, number of smokes per day and drinks per week. Those findings were cross-checked physical characteristics including heart rate and cholesterol level, diseases suffered including mental illness and diabetes. The scientists correlated those results with specific genes suspected in various types of substance abuse. They found more than 400 locations in the genome and at least 566 variants within these locations that influence smoking and alcohol use.

7. Relapse

I know many in sobriety who relapsed multiple times but eventually got and stayed sober. I was in treatment with Clyde, who was an elderly and wealthy man in his 38th time either going up to the door and running away or staying in a treatment facility. This time he stayed and got sober. His story – true, by the way – shows that anyone, regardless of how many times they go back out, can get clean and stay sober.

Almost everyone in recovery has experienced a relapse, according to the National Institute of Drug Abuse. Addiction is a relapsing disease, and some like me have been extremely lucky in not having to go back out. There is a user in me and all of us no matter how long I've been sober. I've witnessed several men who had 20-plus years of sobriety who, on a whim, tasted a beer. One guy kept drinking and ended up in a hospital a couple days later with tubes down his throat.

I'm also at risk, so I honor recovery programs that call for daily maintenance of what we learned in early recovery – take care of myself, apologize for anything stupid I do, stay honest about myself and my behavior. And eat well, get enough sleep, and stay in contact with people. I go to meetings to be with people and soak up their courage.

There are three stages to relapse – emotional, mental and physical. The emotional stage is marked by negative feelings, like "What am I doing here?" and "This ain't working for me," underlaid with anger, moodiness and anxiety. Thoughts of using can again creep in.

The mental stage involves romanticizing the drug use, euphorically recalling the good drinking times, and often depressive thoughts of guilt, worthlessness, and irritability. Thoughts of using get serious.

The physical stage is the "Fuck it" excuse to shuck it all. Most who go back to using find, especially after some sobriety time, that their drug and alcohol use had only gotten worse. Many don't make it back and die some terrible way, but many do. Badly spanked by their experience, they come back in the door ashamed but so happy to have survived and ready to do the work.

8. Relapse Data

I couldn't find statistics on relapse rates for alcoholics and drug addicts and how many came back to fight harder for recovery. I did find the following numbers from the 2017 National Survey on Drug Use and Health of those suffering from a substance use disorder:

• 38% of American adults abused illicit drugs.

• One of every eight adults struggled with alcohol.

• Million American adults also suffered from both a mental health disorder.

• 4 % of children aged 12-17 (992,000 kids).

• About 5.1 million young adults aged 18-25, or 1 in 7.

• Over age 26: 13.6 million, or 6.4 %.

• Age 65 and older: more than 1 million.

• About 9.4% of men and 5.2 % of women age 12 and older.

• Whites: 7.7%, African Americans: 6.8%, Hispanics or Latinos: 6.6%

Here are some statistics on other addictions:

• Gambling: 2.6% or nearly 10 million Americans have a gambling addiction problem. Those 16 to 24 show the most susceptibility, according to the North American Foundation for Gambling Addiction Help are addicts, according to the American Society of Addiction Medicine.

• Sex: There are approximately 18 -24 million Americans who are sex addicts, according to the American Society of Addiction Medicine. Whether it is an addiction or compulsive behavior is still being discussed. About 80% of sex addicts – 8% men, 3% women -- also have another type of addiction, and alcohol and drugs heighten their pleasure.

• Food: There are about 70 million food-addicted adults, according to David Kessler, former commissioner of the U.S. Food and Drug Administration. This addiction occurs in 7% of women and 3% in men.

9. Grief

Psychiatrist Elisabeth Kubler-Ross developed the 5 Stages of Grief, which have been widely accepted. They are: denial, anger, bargaining, depression, and acceptance.

What follows are summaries of research results from various sources:

a. The Journal of NeuroImage: New research suggests that people who never get over their loss, who never "let go," may activate neurons in the reward centers of the brain, possibly giving these memories addiction-like properties.

b. Old Vineyard Behavioral Health Services: Many associate childhood traumas with child abuse, but there are others – tendency to become dependent on alcohol or drugs. neglect, loss of a parent, witnessing domestic or other physical violence, or a parent suffering from mental illness.

c. Those who experience such things during childhood have shown an increased tendency to become dependent on alcohol or drugs. They may also develop behavior addictions such as compulsive eating and compulsive sexual behavior. About two-thirds of all addicts experienced such trauma. Many turn to substance abuse as solution to the pain of the past.

d. American Academy of Child and Adolescent Psychiatry: (For children), a parent who died was essential to the stability of the child's world – anger is a natural reaction. After a parent dies, many children will act younger than they are… and show anger towards the surviving family members … And younger children frequently believe they are the cause of what happens around them.

e. St. Jude's Children Research Hospital: Men turn inward rather than express outwardly. They are less likely to cry, express them-selves verbally, or openly discuss grief with others. Many men do not seek conversation to process their loss…and men tend to want to move past the loss instead of expressing their pain … Men might cope by distraction through physical exercise, working more, or isolating themselves. Women talk with others to process their feelings of loss.

10. Bill Wilson - AA Grapevine, January 1958 (His letter in response to correspondence from an older member earlier in the 1950's)

> "I think that many oldsters who have put our AA "booze cure" to severe but successful tests still find they often lack emo-tional sobriety. Perhaps they will be the spearhead for the next major development in AA, the development of much more real maturity and balance (which is to say, humility) in our re-lations with ourselves, with our fellows, and with God. Those

adolescent urges that so many of us have for top approval, perfect security, and perfect romance, urges quite appropriate to age seventeen, prove to be an impossible way of life when we are at age forty-seven and fifty-seven. Since AA began, I've taken immense wallops in all these areas because of my failure to grow up emotionally and spiritually. My God, how painful it is to keep demanding the impossible, and how very painful to discover, finally, that all along we have had the cart before the horse. Then comes the final agony of seeing how awfully wrong we have been, but still finding ourselves unable to get off the emotional merry-go-round. How to translate a right mental conviction into a right emotional result, and so into easy, happy and good living. Well, that's not only the neurotic's problem, it's the problem of life itself for all of us who have got to the point of real willingness to hew to right principles in all of our affairs. Even then, as we hew away, peace and joy may still elude us. That's the place so many of us AA oldsters have come to. And it's a hell of a spot, literally. How shall our unconscious, from which so many of our fears, compulsions and phony aspirations still stream, be brought into line with what we actually believe, know and want! How to convince our dumb, raging and hidden 'Mr. Hyde' becomes our main task. I've recently come to believe that this can be achieved. I believe so because I begin to see many benighted ones, folks like you and me, commencing to get results. Last autumn, depression, having no really rational cause at all, almost took me to the cleaners. I began to be scared that I was in for another long chronic spell. Considering the grief I've had with depressions, it wasn't a bright prospect. I kept asking myself "Why can't the twelve steps work to release depression?" By the hour, I stared at the St. Francis Prayer ... "it's better to comfort than to be comforted". Here was the formula, all right, but why didn't it work? Suddenly, I realized what the matter was. My basic flaw had always been dependence, almost absolute dependence, on people or circumstances to supply me with prestige, security, and the like. Failing to get these things according to my perfectionist dreams and specifications, I had fought for them. And when defeat came, so did my depression. There wasn't a chance of making the outgoing love of St. Francis a workable and joyous way of life until these fatal and almost absolute dependencies were cut away. Because I had over the years undergone a little spiritual development, the absolute quality of these frightful dependencies had never before been so starkly revealed. Reinforced by what grace I could secure in prayer, I found I had to exert every ounce of will and action to cut off these faulty emotional dependencies upon people, upon AA, indeed upon any act of circumstance whatsoever. Then only could I be free to love as Francis did. Emotional and instinctual satisfactions, I saw, were really the extra dividends of having love, offering love, and expressing love appropriate to each relation of life. Plainly, I could not avail myself to God's love until I was able to offer it back to Him by loving others as He would have me. And I couldn't possibly do that so long as I was victimized by false dependencies. For my dependence meant demand, a demand for the possession and control of the people and the conditions surrounding me. While those words "absolute dependence" may look like a gimmick, they were the ones that helped to trigger my release into my present degree of stability and quietness of mind, qualities which I am now trying to consolidate by offering love to others regardless of the return to me. This seems to be the primary healing circuit: an outgoing love of God's creation and His people, by means of which we avail ourselves of His love for us. It is most clear that the real current can't flow until our paralyzing dependencies are broken, and broken at depth. Only then can we possibly have a glimmer of what adult love really is. Spiritual calculus, you say? Not a bit of it. Watch any AA of six months working with a new Twelfth Step case. If the case says "To the devil with you," the Twelfth Stepper only smiles and turns to another case. He doesn't feel frustrated or rejected. If his next case responds, and in turn starts to give love and attention to other alcoholics, yet gives none back to him, the sponsor is happy about it anyway. He still doesn't feel rejected; he rejoices that his one-time prospect is sober and happy. And if his next following case turns out in later time to be his best friend (or romance) then the sponsor is most joyful. But he well knows that his happiness is a by-product -- the extra dividend of giving without any demand for a return. The really stabilizing thing for him was having and offering love to that strange drunk on his doorstep. That was Francis at work, powerful and practical, minus dependency and minus demand. In the first six months of my own sobriety, I worked hard with many alcoholics. Not a one responded. Yet this work kept me sober. It wasn't a question of those alcoholics giving me anything. My stability came out of trying to give, not out of demanding that I receive. Thus, I think it can work out with emotional sobriety. If we examine every disturbance we have, great or small, we will find at the root of it some unhealthy dependency and its consequent unhealthy demand. Let us, with God's help, continually surrender these hobbling demands. Then we can be set free to live and love; we may then be able to Twelfth Step ourselves and others into emotional sobriety.

Of course, I haven't offered you a really new idea – only a gimmick that has started to unhook several of my own hexes at depth. Nowadays, my brain no longer races compulsively in neither elation, grandiosity nor depression. I have been given a quiet place in bright sunshine.

--**Bill Wilson**

11. Science

The science of quantum mechanics has revealed that everything is made of energy. Remember Einstein's famous equation – Energy equals mass times the speed of light squared ($E=mc2$). It's always intrigued me that when I'm in a bad mood I somehow find more fuel for that mood, but when I'm feeling good, everything I see and do energizes my happiness. It seems to me that science may eventually have something to say about this. I believe it, and others do, too.

The Law of Attraction states that everything in the universe is energy, and everything is connected to everything else. *The Lucid Dream Manifesto, reprinted in 2006, puts it this way: Energy attracts like energy. You do not attract your desires by what you think but by what you feel. Energy is vibration, and you attract those things that you are in vibrational resonance with. Your vibration is your feeling.*

Suggested Reading

These are books that helped me to know myself, understand my past, and grow up to live a wonderful life. All of them are readily available in bookstores and libraries.

The Solace of Fierce Landscapes by Belden C. Lane

"Fierce Landscapes and the Indifference of God" by Belden C. Lane (article found online)

The Road Less Traveled by M. Scott Peck

The Prince of Tides and *The Great Santini* by Pat Conroy

The River Why by David James Duncan

The Artist's Way by Julia Cameron

The Wild Edge of Sorrow by Francis Weller

Any book by Claudia Black

Zen and the Art of Motorcycle Maintenance by Robert M. Pirsig

Some books by recovering authors:

Drinking: A Love Story by Caroline Knapp

Blackout: Remembering the Thing I Drank to Forget by Sarah Hepola

The Unexpected Joy of Being Sober by Catherine Gray